NATURAL HEALING FOR

BACK PAIN

NATURAL HEALING FOR

BACK PAIN

SIMPLE AND SAFE COMPLEMENTARY
FIRST-AID AND SELF-HELP TREATMENTS

LEON CHAITOW ND DO

CONTENTS

CHAPTER ONE

UNDERSTANDING BACK PAIN

Back pain affects about 75 percent of the population at some time during their adult lives, so the chances are you will already have experienced, or are likely to experience, backache severe enough to require you to stop, or reduce, your normal activities for a while.

PREVENTING BACK PAIN

Greater detail on the people most likely to develop backache can be found on pages 12–13. Half of all cases of backache start suddenly—often caused by bending. About half of these involve disk changes ("slipped disk"), while most others involve either muscular or joint problems (see pages 12–13, 18–19). The other half start slowly; symptoms may come and go, or gradually progress until the backache is severe.

In many cases there are inborn biomechanical reasons for backache, and these are examined on pages 15. In others the causes lie in habits of use, posture, working, and recreational behavior (see pages 16–17). The ways in which the wonderfully engineered body slowly adapts to the multiple stress factors which affect all off us are discussed on pages 20–21 and emotional causes on pages 22–23. Finally, pages 24–25 show how bad breathing habits can lead to back pain.

Why are some afflicted by backache and not others, and why are humans prone to backache? Few animals are—apart from overweight dogs and unnaturally stressed racehorses. Part of the answer lies in our upright posture, which strains the back unless we are perfectly balanced. Therapies such as the Alexander Technique teach good posture (see page 70)—something we seldom see in modern human beings!

The demands on the back are often enormous. Consider the compound stresses of:

- Regularly recurring occupational strains such as bending, sitting awkwardly, long periods of standing, and strain-inducing movements.

- Wearing physiologically stressful footwear (high heels in particular, and platform shoes).

- Fitting our variously shaped bodies into mass-produced and poorly designed furniture and driving seats.

- Habits such as sitting cross-legged, standing with the weight on one leg, and slumped posture.

Consider also a daily routine which may include:

- Sleeping on too soft a bed, with pillows which are too high, pushing the body into a strained position even while resting.

- Stooping over a uniform-height sink.

- Adapting anything but uniform body sizes to standardly shaped and sized transportation.

- Work, study, or leisure positions which may involve carrying, lengthy periods of standing, or sitting at ill-designed desks.

POSTURE IN GORILLA AND MAN

POSTURE AND BODY STRUCTURE IN GORILLA AND MAN

The gradual adoption of an upright stance has turned the human spine from a perfect cantilevered bridge into an unstable skyscraper.

Adaption to upright posture has not yet been fully achieved, and the high incidence of backache is one major result. Even the partially adapted gorilla has a more stable spine than ours.

Unless we are perfectly balanced, upright posture puts enormous strain on the back. Methods like the Alexander Technique are intended to prevent the strain.

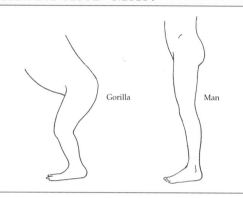

Gorilla   Man

Muscular tensions produced by the emotions of the day which reflect the demands of our lives and our struggles to cope with these.

And all this may be undertaken in high heels, in a habitually one-sided manner, and with a slouch or stoop. Is it any wonder humans have been described as "biped animals with a backache"? Even in our leisure we have bizarre stresses imposed on the body by:

- One-sided sports like tennis, golf, and baseball.

- Repetitive activities which may also stress parts of the body, like weight training, skiing, athletics, aerobics, rowing, and gymnastics.

- Sheer lack of exercise—inactivity leading to weak muscle tone and poor spinal support.

Other reasons for backache range from injury to diseases such as rheumatoid arthritis and osteoporosis. In summary, overuse, abuse, misuse and disuse are the most common causes of backache.

What's to be done?
Our task in any case of backache is to identify and reduce or eliminate those causes which we can do something about through better posture, less repetitive strain, improved use of the body during daily activities, reduced referred pain from emotional overload and so on.

Where causes cannot be dealt with, and changes have taken place in the muscles and joints, our task is to offer solutions which can improve matters or, at the very least, prevent things from getting worse, by:

- Stretching what is tight and restricted.

- Toning what is weak.

- Reeducating the individual in how to use the body efficiently and safely.

These approaches—removing causes, and safely encouraging normal function—are the ideal for prevention as well as relief of backache and are the aims of this book.

THE INCIDENCE OF BACK PAIN

Why hasn't evolution prepared our backs for lifting?

Shouldn't we have become used to bending and lifting strains over the past hundreds of thousands of years since our early ancestors stopped walking on all fours?

Research by anthropologists suggests hunter-gatherers (around half-a-million people still live this way in South America, Africa and Australia, so we can study their habits) bend or carry things around 50 times daily. In modern Western society, with all its labor-saving gadgets, the number of times people bend and carry can often amount to an incredible 5,000 times daily! That is a 100 percent increase.

We have hardly adapted to this and are unlikely to for a long, long time. In nonindustrialized societies posture tends to be much better than in Western society. Put simply, muscle tone is better, use of the body is more efficient, and backache is much rarer. We can learn a lot from this example.

BACK PAIN: WHO IS MOST AT RISK?

- People in occupations which involve lifting are at risk, with miners, dockers, and workers in heavy industry (steel and so on), and the building trades being exposed to repetitive heavy strains.

- Professional dancers are at high risk, along with athletes, especially if they engage in contact sport.

- Drivers (bus, taxi, truck, and private) as well airline pilots and flight crews.

- Anyone regularly bending and lifting is at risk, even if what they lift is light. Examples include people stacking supermarket shelves and warehouse workers, airline attendants, nursery school teachers, nurses, physical therapists, osteopaths, chiropractors, and massage therapists!

- Farmers, foresters, horticulturists, and gardeners (domestic or commercial) all face numerous hazards which can stress their backs.

- Assembly-line workers, plumbers, carpenters, and painters all risk injury from repetitive tasks, as do professionals such as dentists and surgeons.

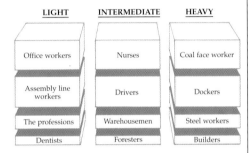

LIGHT	INTERMEDIATE	HEAVY
Office workers	Nurses	Coal face worker
Assembly line workers	Drivers	Dockers
The professions	Warehousemen	Steel workers
Dentists	Foresters	Builders

- People who stand most of the day, such as store workers, hairdressers, and lecturers/teachers risk back problems if their posture is not excellent.

- People in sedentary occupations face lower—but still significant—risks.

- Office workers sitting at a computer terminal for hours on end face hazards from ill-designed workstations and chairs.

- Military personnel of many types are involved in stresses which place the back at risk. The list is almost as endless as the variety of occupations.

The cost of backache

For many people the experience of a backache is short-lived; pain often starts suddenly, the back becomes stiff, and movement increasingly difficult and limited for a period of time. After a few days' rest, with or without treatment, no symptoms remain and the backache is only a memory. If this was all that happened in all cases of backache the problem would not warrant the attention we are giving it. Unfortunately, for many others the story is quite different, with pain and dysfunction lasting weeks or months or even years. The cost goes beyond the pain experienced; it is measured both in lost working time (welfare benefits seldom make up for lost earnings) and the cost of treatments.

There is also the cost to society of tens of millions of lost working hours. In the UK, for example, over 35 million working days are lost each year through back problems alone, and in the United States (and other countries such as Sweden) back pain is the largest single reason for time off work in people under 45 years of age.

The nature of back ache

Pain in the back can result from:

- Muscles going into spasm because they suffer acute or chronic strain—which irritates the nerves which pass through them.

- A disk may herniate (bulge) so that the "pulp" from the disk presses on nerves and local muscles go into protective spasm.

- Facet joints between vertebrae (see page 18) or sacroiliac joints in the pelvis can be injured and inflamed (by twisting, jarring movements, for example). Nerves from these tissues can become irritated and painful.

The pain which is felt in the back is actually recorded in the brain, and scientific research has shown ways of interrupting or confusing the reception of the pain messages by "closing the gate" to them. This features in some of the self-treatment methods described on pages 58-59.

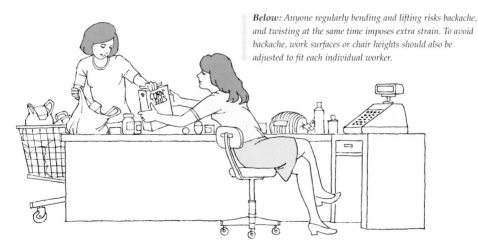

Below: Anyone regularly bending and lifting risks backache, and twisting at the same time imposes extra strain. To avoid backache, work surfaces or chair heights should also be adjusted to fit each individual worker.

CAUSES OF BACK PAIN

The cause of some back pain lies in systemic conditions affecting the whole body, and not local back problems. It is not in the scope of this book to deal with the needs of people with systemic conditions such as fibromyalgia (fibrositis) or arthritis, who require specialized advice and care. Our concerns focus on bio-mechanical forms of back pain, such as that which occurs when we bend or lift awkwardly.

When we bend to lift or reach something, the hinge joints of the knees and hips should lower us toward the floor, with the lower back staying relatively straight. Once we start to use the spine as a hinge, a degree of strain is imposed on what is essentially a weight-bearing structure, not designed to bend and flex. When we contort that way we stretch and twist muscles as well as imposing enormous stress loads on the inter-vertebral disks (see pages 18–19)

Muscle strain

If muscles are already compromised through previous or repetitive strain, or from lack of exercise, a slight degree of additional stress—a sudden movement, a shifting of the load being lifted or a cough or sneeze while stooping—might induce a protective muscle spasm. Tense muscles have two major features:

- A slow but constant buildup of fluid metabolic wastes in the body of the muscle.

- A reduction in the ability of fresh, oxygenated blood to flow freely into and through the muscle to nourish it and to carry away wastes.

A combination of retained wastes and reduced oxygenation makes muscles feel uncomfortable—see how long you keep your fist clenched without feeling an ache and eventually a pain! Such muscles are also far more likely to "cramp" or go into spasm than are well-oxygenated and well-drained tissues.

Over time, weeks rather than months, stressed muscles will adapt by replacing elastic fibers with more inelastic, tough ones. This makes the muscle more able to bear loads but far less able to resist any sudden demands which call for elasticity. Stability is gained at the expense of vulnerability.

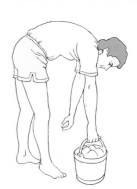

LIFTING

Right: *When picking up heavy burdens, the back should be kept straight, and the leg muscles should take the weight of the object. This protects the back muscles and the spine itself, which should not function as a hinge.*

Far right: *The back is a weight-bearing structure and is not designed to bend and flex. Bending from the hips to pick up a weight puts enormous stress on the back. It strains both the muscles and the intervertebral disks.*

Two types of muscle

Recent research has shown not all muscles are the same. "Phasic" muscles move whatever they are attached to, enabling us, for instance, to pick up a cup to drink from.

"Postural" muscles stabilize the structures (bones) to which they are attached. Your arm could not lift the cup if your shoulder were not stabilized by postural muscles.

All muscles have what are called fast-twitch and slow-twitch fibers. In phasic muscles there are more of the fast-twitch type and in postural muscles more of the slow-twitch type.

This knowledge is important in understanding the causes of back problems because when muscles are stressed (by bad posture or repetitive use, for example) postural and phasic muscles behave quite differently.

- Phasic muscles under stress become weaker ("inhibited").

- Postural muscles under stress become shorter and tighter.

This has major implications for backs. When you lift a cup, the action is a smooth one. As your arm bends to bring the cup to your mouth, the muscles on the front of the arm contract, while those on the back relax. Otherwise the muscles would fight each other. This happens because of a control mechanism called reciprocal inhibition. A contracting muscle will inhibit or weaken its antagonist (the muscle which performs the opposite movement), allowing smooth movement.

When a muscle is constantly tight—as in a low back stressed by postural or occupational strains, the opposite muscles (the abdominals) become weak and the abdomen sags. How many people can you spot with taut lower back muscles which arch their lower backs, and with weak, sagging abdomens? Most will have backache.

INBORN BALANCES

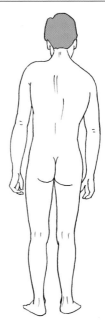

FUNCTIONAL/POSTURAL STRESS

Anyone with one leg shorter than the other (most people have one leg slightly longer than the other) has a range of muscle compensations taking place. A sequence occurs in which some muscles become shorter and others become slacker (see pages 20-21). Whatever the causes, whether a short leg or a postural habit, or a job which calls for repeated movement, the end result is the same—some muscles shorten while others become weaker. These imbalances produce many cases of backache, and this book offers safe solutions to such problems through stretching and toning and, above all, through better habits.

MISUSE, OVERUSE, AND ABUSE AS CAUSES OF BACK PAIN

Sitting or standing badly or repeatedly stressing and contorting the body generates the muscle imbalances discussed on pages 14–15, leading to muscle weakness and shortness. At the same time local changes in muscles lead to extremely sensitive tissues, called myofascial trigger points (see page 58-59), where nerve structures become overreactive and irritable. These not only hurt when they are touched or moved, but also refer pain to target areas some distance away. Trigger points produce a good deal of the pain felt by backache sufferers, and we will examine ways of easing them by self-help later on.

Sitting as a cause of backache

The firmness or softness of a seat, and its angle and height relative to the sitter's leg length, as well as to the working surface, all have a direct influence on health. The type of job an individual does and the way the equipment or material they are working with is set out are also important factors in back stress. An ideal sitting position is one in which:

- The seat is tilted slightly forward—10–15 degrees is adequate.

- Either the feet are flat on the floor,

- Or the knees are supported on a padded surface, in a "kneeler" type chair.

- The thighs are at an angle of between 110 and 130 degrees to the trunk.

A forward-tilting seat can be achieved by placing a wedge-shaped cushion on the seat or by an adjustable mechanism; both methods produce an ideal sitting position. Sitting on an unadjustable seat for hours can bring major stresses to the back, as it encourages a tendency to slump; this is reduced when good seating is provided. Correct prescription eye glasses or contact lenses help to correct the habit of twisting the head to one side.

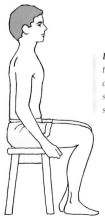

Left: A chair should be adjusted to the individual: the feet should be flat on the floor and the knees should be supported. The back should be kept straight while stting.

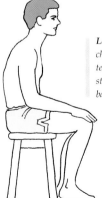

Left: Sitting on an unadjustable chair for many hours can encourage a tendency to slump, which is a major stress on the back and often leads to back pain.

HIGH HEELS AND BACKACHE

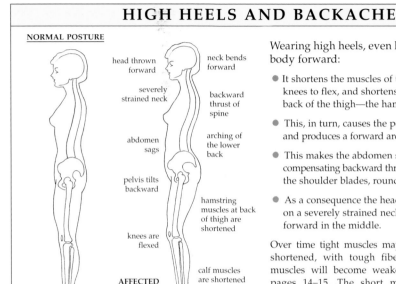

NORMAL POSTURE

head thrown forward

severely strained neck

abdomen sags

pelvis tilts backward

knees are flexed

AFFECTED POSTURE

neck bends forward

backward thrust of spine

arching of the lower back

hamstring muscles at back of thigh are shortened

calf muscles are shortened

Wearing high heels, even low ones, throws the body forward:

- It shortens the muscles of the calf, causing the knees to flex, and shortens the muscles at the back of the thigh—the hamstrings.

- This, in turn, causes the pelvis to tilt backward and produces a forward arching of the lower back.

- This makes the abdomen sag and produces a compensating backward thrust of the spine between the shoulder blades, rounding the shoulders.

- As a consequence the head is thrown forward on a severely strained neck which bends forward in the middle.

Over time tight muscles may become permanently shortened, with tough fibers developing. Other muscles will become weakened as discussed on pages 14–15. The short muscles could require extensive manual treatment and/or self-help stretching to help normalize them.

Workstations as a cause of backache

The average head weighs between 12 and 15 pounds, and the neck and shoulder muscles are stressed if it is held forward of the neck. This often happens in desk-work situations.

- Reading material should be approximately 10 to 20 degrees below the horizontal line of vision, as on a reading stand. A flat desk or table encourages neck-craning; this stresses the upper back via the muscles supporting and moving the head.

- To avoid repeatedly twisting the neck, work should be in front, not to the side. Work should be 12 to 24 inches from the eyes.

Standing posture as a cause of backache

Poor posture is a common cause of backache but good posture is impossible when there are imbalances between the major postural muscles until shortened muscles are stretched and weak muscles strengthened. Ideally the head should balance on the neck, with the crown of the head (not the front) the highest point, and the neck should "lengthen" rather than thrusting forward.

Sleep posture

Ideally we should sleep on our side on a firm but not hard bed with a single pillow to prevent neck tilting. Sleeping on your front twists the neck. Sleeping on the back is safe if the neck and head are supported but not thrust forward.

JOINT AND DISK PROBLEMS

"Slipped disk"

The spine is important to the human body to:

● House a canal, along which runs the vital cord which carries the link between the brain and the rest of the body. The spinal cord makes function and movement possible.

● To provide a central connecting structure for the body, which enables us to stand, walk, and move freely.

● To carry the weight of the head and the upper trunk.

In humans this bony bridge is carried vertically rather than horizontally, exposing the spine to the additional problem of the forces of gravity. The bones of the spine are separated by wonderfully constructed pads—the disks. These:

● Protect the spinal cord.
● Help spread the load.
● Act as shock absorbers against the jars and jolts our body encounters daily.

Each disk consists of a tough, outer cartilaginous ring, enclosing an inner pulpy, jellylike, substance. Each disk attaches firmly to the vertebrae above and below it. When injury or wear and tear cause a gap, tear, or herniation (bulge) in this cartilaginous outer surface, the pulpy material may protrude and press on nerves emerging from the spine as well as local soft tissues, bringing acute, often agonizing, pain and spasm. This is commonly known as a "slipped disk."

Sometimes a disk slowly degenerates, and becomes narrower, and a less efficient shock absorber. Stiffness, loss of full mobility and pain could then result. The possible results include a ruptured disk or degenerated disk, but neither is inevitable, and many people reach old age without either occuring.

Disks cannot slip but they can herniate—and once this has happened the disk cannot be "put back," although a slow healing is usually possible as the body reabsorbs the protruding pulp. Appropriate treatment to ease spasm, stretch tightened local soft tissues, strengthen

SWOLLEN FACET JOINT

NORMAL FACET JOINT

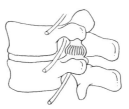

SWOLLEN FACET JOINT

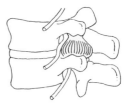

Above: Much back pain results partly from damaged facet joints, and it is these which chiropractors and osteopaths may manipulate when trying to normalize restricted spinal movement.

weak musculature and mobilize restricted joints can speed this healing process along, especially when it is combined with suitable reeducation and self-help measures.

In some cases, however, where the protruding pulp presses directly onto the nerves, surgery may be the only option. To be successful this must be followed by intensive physical therapy to rehabilitate the region.

The main way disks become progressively damaged, preparing them for an acute herniation, is repetitive postural insults such as bending incorrectly, slouching, and generally using the spine in ways for which it was not designed (see previous pages).

Spinal and pelvic joint strains

If the spine were supported only by a series of disks it would be unstable. However, a series of bony contacts between each vertebra and the ones above and below it—called facet joints—provide extra strength. They form the back portion of the outer covering of the spinal cord itself, and create a space through which nerves pass to and from the spinal cord, carrying all the information which keeps us functioning.

The facet joints provide safety and support. Along with ligaments and muscles, they prevent the spine from rotating too far, and they absorb much of the force of jars and strains.

When injuries overwhelm the disk's shock-absorbing capacity, the facet joints can be damaged, bruising and irritating them, leading to both local and reflex pain in the associated soft-tissue structures.

Much back pain results partly from damaged facet joints, and it is these which chiropractors and osteopaths may manipulate when trying to normalize restricted spinal movement.

Treatment which frees the supporting soft tissues can also assist in correcting back problems associated with facet joint irritation. Suitable self-help exercises which encourage flexibility and mobility (see pages 32–39) can assist in keeping the facet joints in good working order.

Pelvic problems and backache

The spine stands on the flat base of the sacral bone, which itself is "wedged" between the huge pelvic "wing-bones," the ilia. Anything which causes the sacrum to be tilted—such as a short leg, shortened hamstring muscle, or restriction at the sacroiliac joint—will make the spine slant to one side instead of being straight, placing excessive stress on the disks and facet joints, as well as on the supporting muscles, leading inevitably to pain.

We cannot have a healthy, pain-free spine without having a well-functioning pelvis—and this calls for the muscles which attach to it being in a balanced state—not excessively tight or weak. The exercises on pages 32–39 will encourage this.

LUMBAR VERTEBRA AND PELVIS

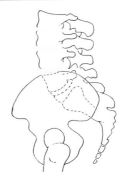

Above: We cannot have a healthy, pain-free spine without having a well-functioning pelvis—and this calls for the muscles attached to it being in a balanced state—not excessively tight or weak.

MUSCULAR IMBALANCES AND BACKACHE

When postural muscles tighten and shorten because of chronic stress—possibly because of inborn variations such as one leg being shorter than the other, or overuse or injury—the muscles which perform the opposite movements to these stressed muscles (called the antagonists) become "inhibited" or weaker. This can cause chain reactions of muscular imbalance in which whole areas of the body are put under strain.

"The Lower Crossed Syndrome"
The muscles at the front of the hip (such as psoas) may become overactive and short while their antagonists at the back (the gluteals) sometimes become weaker.

At the same time, the muscles of the lower back, which support the spine (the erector spinae), may become overactive and short, while their antagonist group (the abdominal muscles) become weak.

The picture which then emerges, sometimes called "the lower crossed syndrome," is one of imbalance and stress for the low back.

This alters not only the mechanical position of the back, but also the way the body moves, placing even more stress on the area.

For example, when we walk one leg goes forward and the other is momentarily behind the trunk—this is called "extension" of the back leg. Leg extension should be produced by contraction of the gluteals working together with the hamstring muscles of the leg. If either of these is weaker than it should be—as the gluteals would be in the syndrome described above—other muscles have to take on their task. In this example it is the low back muscles which would overwork every time a step was taken. This

would make them even tighter, which would lead to even weaker action by the abdominal muscles, producing a sagging abdomen as well as low-back pain. The chain reaction of tightness, weakness and inappropriate activity is an all-too-common picture, which progresses up the body to yet another syndrome.

"The Upper Crossed Syndrome"
With the lower crossed syndrome pattern we see an arched lower back and a sagging abdomen.

● This causes the area between the shoulder blades to be carried farther back than is normal and, consequently, the shoulders and head to be thrust forward, putting strain on particular postural muscles—particularly the pectoral muscles in front of the upper chest, and the upper trapezius muscles, which lie between the base of the neck and the shoulder.

● As these tighten and shorten (see pages 14–15) their antagonists become weaker—in this case the muscles between the shoulder blades (lower trapezius), as well as the flexor muscles of the neck.

In the "upper crossed syndrome," the shoulders are rounded, the head is in front of the neck and the chin pokes forward.

This leads inevitably to aching in the upper back and neck. The shoulders will also ache because the shoulder blades are not where they should be—they have drifted upward and sideways, giving a slumped, round-shouldered appearance.

Another link has formed in a chain reaction of tightness-weakness-imbalance.

It is easy to determine whether this syndrome is operating by feeling whether particular muscles are working when they shouldn't be.

POSTURAL MUSCLE IMBALANCES

LOWER CROSSED SYNDROME

The muscles at the front of the hip (such as psoas) may become overactive and short while their antagonists at the back (the gluteals) sometimes become weaker.

With the lower-crossed-syndrome pattern we see an arched low back and a sagging abdomen.

UPPER CROSSED SYNDROME

In the "upper crossed syndrome," the shoulders are rounded, the head is in front of the neck, and the chin pokes forward. This leads inevitably to aching in the upper back and neck. The shoulders will also ache because the shoulder blades are not where they should be.

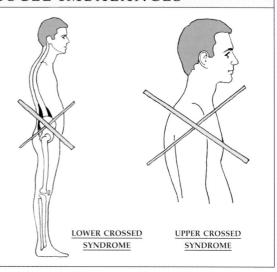

LOWER CROSSED
SYNDROME

UPPER CROSSED
SYNDROME

Just as some muscles were used inappropriately for walking when the lower-crossed pattern was evident, we see a similar imbalance in swinging the arm during walking when the upper crossed syndrome is present.

When we walk one arm goes forward and the other backward. The action of carrying the arm back should NOT involve the upper trapezius. To determine if this is happening, take your left hand (say) across your chest and rest it over the area between your neck and your right shoulder. Then take your right arm backward, as you would if you were walking. You should not feel any activity, nor any contraction in the muscle under your hand.

If you do feel a contraction, the muscle is over-active, working when it should not be working. Because it is a postural muscle it will become shorter and tighter, and produce not only local pain but also can produce pain at a distance (in the head and face usually) because of trigger points which will develop in it.

These patterns of dysfunction—lower and upper syndromes—lead to breathing restrictions (how can the ribs move properly when the shoulders are rounded?) and even more stress on postural muscles, creating greater chance of back pain.

The solution

Part of it is to begin to normalize the postural muscles which have shortened, and in later sections of the book we will examine the muscles one by one and offer specific self-help exercises to help normalize them. This will allow their antagonists to strengthen again and balance can be restored. Of course if the causes of the strain on the muscles—poor posture perhaps—is not also corrected, the problem will come back.

EMOTIONAL INFLUENCES

In some cases emotional problems have been "locked away" in the body, and the backache or neck pain a person feels is not entirely physical in nature, but has its roots in their emotions. The medical term for this is somatization. The pain is no less real—but it does mean a purely physical approach to treating it may not be completely successful. The causes of the symptoms have to be treated if they are to be completely removed.

Depression

Look at the drawing of the person who has a "depressed" posture on page 23. The weight of the world is carried on his shoulders; he cannot look the world in the eye, he gazes constantly down or avoids eye contact with others, and his shoulders are stooped. He looks the way he feels—heavy and burdened.

There is a cartoon in the *Snoopy* series in which Charlie Brown is standing like this, and is saying to a friend, "If you're going to get any pleasure out of being depressed, this is how you have to stand.' This black humor makes a point—our posture says a good deal about how we feel.

As we have seen in previous pages, if muscles are used in ways which place them under stress and tension for prolonged periods, they will change in their structure and function:

- Muscles which shorten (postural muscles) will, over time, not just be tense but will develop fibrous bands and will not be able to relax in the way a tense muscle can; they will need physical treatment such as stretching before they return to normal.

- Weak phasic muscles will need to have the causes of their weakness corrected (their tense and tight antagonists will need to be normalized, for example), as well as being toned up by exercise to return to normal.

- In addition to whole muscle changes, local trigger points (pages 58-59) will develop and these will cause pain both in the muscles housing them and at a distance, often in the back. This pattern can be produced just as easily by emotional tension as by injury, overuse or postural stress. Over time the person who stands in a "depressed slump" will be held in that position by the changes in their muscles even after their depression has ended.

Anxiety

Equally distinctive is the posture and pattern of use of anxious individuals. They commonly hold themselves in an "attack-defense" posture—hunched shoulders, jutting head and clenched teeth. The shoulders give a clue to what is actually happening, because in an anxiety state the breathing pattern alters.

There is a tendency for the upper chest to be used instead of the diaphragm, giving excessive work to the muscles which link the upper ribs to the neck. These should only work as breathing muscles when we exert ourselves, such as by running. They are postural muscles and as such their main task is to support the neck. When they are overused because of anxiety they shorten, and as they shorten they stress the neck and upper back and produce a variety of symptoms, including:

- Headaches
- Neck pain
- Shoulder ache
- Upper backache
- Chest pain
- Increased anxiety

POSTURE AND MOOD

DEPRESSED POSTURE   **GOOD POSTURE**   **ANXIETY POSTURE**

Far Left: *A person with a depressed posture is easily recognized. The weight of the world is upon them; they cannot look the world in the eye; they gaze constantly down.*

Middle left: *Good posture can be encouraged through relaxation training, meditation, and physical exercise, which help relax the body and defuse any negative feelings.*

Left: *Equally distinctive is the posture of anxious individuals. They commonly hold themselves in an attack posture—hunched shoulders, jutting head and clenched teeth.*

This completes the circle and keeps the disturbed breathing pattern going. This pattern of disturbance is common in people with chronic fatigue who overuse muscles, are underoxygenated, and develop a series of symptoms directly linked to the pattern described above.

The answer to such problems is necessarily complex. The tight and short structures must be normalized by treatment and exercise, and breathing must be retrained. The original anxiety may also need to be dealt with, although it may be long gone, having left the individual with unconscious habits of breathing, and all the repercussions described above.

Other emotional states

All emotions reflect to some extent in our muscles. Whatever the feelings, we inevitably reflect them in our bodies. Anger is often "held" in arm muscles, fear can affect leg and abdominal muscles, and frustration can be held in the leg and back muscles. If we hold these emotions for lengthy periods, physical changes will occur and we will develop long-term symptoms.

Methods which relax the body and defuse the negative feelings are likely to help; these include relaxation training, meditation, and physical exercise. Counseling or psychotherapy can also be useful for some individuals.

BAD BREATHING HABITS

Many people are upper-chest breathers, putting a great deal of strain on their muscles and joints, especially those associated with the middle and upper parts of the chest and back.

Breathing is a function which is both automatic and under our direct control; we can easily hold our breath but we cannot ask our heart to stop beating or our liver to stop working. Breathing is also a function which has a very close link with our emotions, and it seems many people tend toward bad breathing habits from a very early age, especially if they do not get enough exercise. This can cause:

● Fatigue.

● A lack of oxygen circulating the body because breathing is too shallow.

● Overuse of muscles which should not be working.

● Increased anxiety (aggravated by the tendency to breathe out too much carbon dioxide).

● Neck, shoulder, and backache.

When we run it is perfectly normal for the muscles which link the upper ribs and the neck to become active—so that we can take in more fresh air and breathe out more used air, as we exert ourselves. These muscles are called "accessory" breathing muscles, and are meant to be used in this way only during exertion. Unfortunately many of us learn bad breathing habits when quite young and over breathe, or become "upper chest breathers," in response to situations other than when we are exerting ourselves. This often occurs when we feel anxious or frightened.

How the muscles and joints are affected

This pattern of breathing causes a great deal of extra work, not just for the muscles which are overworking but also for the joints associated with the bones to which the muscles are anchored. (Muscles have to have attachments on bone or they could not pull and push our limbs when we want to work or walk.)

● Overuse of certain muscles leads to a series of "imbalances" in which some become overtight and others overweak.

● As explained on pages 14-15, the process of "reciprocal inhibition" occurs when some muscles tighten and the opposite muscle becomes "inhibited."

This means when we overbreathe and overuse certain muscles they develop extra "tone" or tension, and their opposing muscles will at the same time become weaker. The postural stress pattern which emerges from this progression of events leads to serious back problems.

Lower-back muscles

Two important low-back muscles are affected by upper-chest breathing, because they both have fibers which merge with the diaphragm. These are the quadratus lumborum and iliopsoas. These muscles lie in the small of the back (quadratus) and on the front of the lower spine

Psoas muscles

Left: If the psoas or quadratus muscles are shortened by upper-chest breathing, a great deal of trouble for the back can be expected.

24

NEGATIVE EFFECTS OF UPPER-CHEST BREATHING

We can now examine the sequence of events which occur when a habit of upper-chest breathing exists. The effect is similar although not as severe as what happens in someone with asthma, who cannot help breathing this way.

1 The muscles of the middle and upper back get progressively tighter as they overwork, with resulting weakness of the muscles of the abdomen (the antagonists).

2 The middle areas of the spine (thoracic spine) will become tense because of the stress to the ribs which connect with it and the muscles which are attached to it.

3 The muscles of the neck and shoulders will also become extremely tense, often leading to the head being held in a way that kinks the neck and pokes the chin forward.

4 The neck itself will become progressively more stiff.

5 The overworked accessory breathing muscles will develop tough fibrotic changes as they respond to the repetitive demands made by unbalanced breathing habits (thousands of times a day). They will also develop trigger points (pages 58-59).

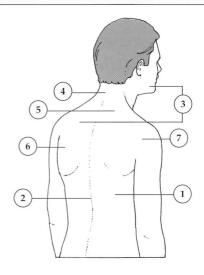

6 Because of these muscular changes the shoulder blades will be held in a different position to normal, so that the shoulders will "round."

7 This strains the muscles of the shoulder and upper back, and the pectoral muscles in the front of the shoulders, resulting in fibrosis, trigger points (pages 58-59), restriction, and, eventually, pain.

(psoas) running to the hip joint. If these muscles become short, a great deal of trouble for the back can be expected. When they are in spasm these muscles produce the crablike, distorted movement associated with "lumbago."

These physical effects of upper-chest breathing are accompanied by significant emotional effects, as this pattern of breathing encourages anxiety as well as being a common result of anxiety.

The answer to the complex problems which can result from imbalanced breathing does not just involve learning how to breathe correctly, although this is essential for long-term recovery and prevention of repetitive recurrence of pain and restriction. The real answer lies in a combination of bodywork, soft-tissue stretching and release, joint mobilization, and removal of trigger points—accompanied by breathing reeducation.

CHAPTER TWO

CURRENT MEDICAL CARE

Diagnostically speaking, this is a golden age for understanding the
mechanics of back problems. Medical workers trying to evaluate and make
sense of the many different diseases and dysfunctions which afflict the
human spine now have a range of tools available.

DIAGNOSIS

Medical workers can view not only the bony structures, but, through the magic of magnetic resonance imaging (MRI) and similar scanning techniques, muscles, tendons, ligaments, soft tissues, and fascia.

For many years X-ray has been a standard diagnostic tool for the back. It remains, together with the newer and safer, if more expensive, technology, the ideal way to see pathology—damage caused by arthritis or disk herniation, or structural and positional changes such as occur after trauma or dislocation. Knowing what has happened is important, but it does not solve the

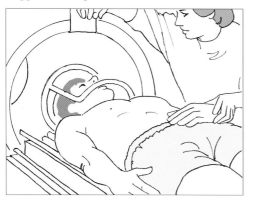

problem. Evidence that there is a disease process such as arthritis or rheumatism associated with a person's back pain *might* guide the doctor or therapist to the best possible course of treatment, but equally this may not yet be entirely clear. However, scan and X-ray results can usually guide therapists and practitioners as to what *not* to do, and to what treatment might be likely to make the situation worse.

Because these tests, some of which are still very expensive, are now available from commercial laboratories as well as many hospitals, they are used widely by orthodox medical personnel as well as by chiropractors, physical therapists, osteopaths, and other manual therapists—if clients are wealthy enough to afford the cost themselves, or if their health insurance covers them for this type of investigation.

Whether or not the evidence from a scan or X-ray shows pathology or structural changes, the doctor or therapist will still need to investigate the problem farther by means of painstaking history-taking, followed by palpation and testing procedures which can provide a much clearer picture of what has happened, or what is happening, and what needs doing.

Left: Through the magic of magnetic resonance imaging the
practitioner can see all the potential areas of pain in the back;
the soft tissues, muscles, tendons, ligaments, and fascia.

These manual and visual tests examine:

- The way individual joints are working.
- The status of muscles (tight, short, weak).
- The presence or absence of active trigger points (see pages 58-59).
- The functional status of whole regions: how they differ from normal or expected behavior.

Today, the diagnostic methods used by doctors and physical therapists differs little from those used by chiropractors and osteopaths; it is the use made of the information which differs so much.

Orthodox treatment of general backache
When it comes to the treatment of backaches, the most common advice offered by most doctors is to rest and take anti-inflammatory drugs and/or painkillers. The value of such approaches should be questioned.

It has been found that patients with backache who go to a medical doctor do not recover as rapidly as those receiving alternative advice and manipulative treatment. Research shows that patients receiving chiropractic or osteopathic care are back at work much faster, and maintain their improvement for much longer, than people who take bed rest and medical drugs for their back problems.

Modern physical therapy has now adopted many of the manipulative methods of alternative back care. However, it tends to use these devices alongside various mechanical aids, such as ultrasound, heat and interferential treatment, and the results are extremely good.

Bed rest has been shown to actually slow down recovery from most back problems, though an acute disk condition does require rest. The use of painkillers and antiinflammatory drugs, while reducing discomfort, also has negative effects, particularly on the digestive system.

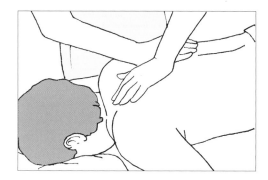

Above: The old prejudices which prevented referral to alternative practitioners and therapists are breaking down, and many medical doctors now suggest manipulative therapy rather than bed rest for backache.

New trends
In some medical settings a tendency is developing for osteopaths and chiropractors to work in a team with physical therapists. The latter concentrate on rehabilitation and retraining, while the former deal with the structural and mechanical problems of backache sufferers. The old prejudices which prevented referral to alternative therapists are breaking down and many doctors now suggest manipulative therapy rather than bed rest for backache.

Acupuncture and trigger point injections
A great many doctors are also now utilizing acupuncture (or are referring patients with pain problems to acupuncturists), and this form of treatment is standard in specialist medical pain control clinics.

In such clinics procaine or xylocaine injections will also be used to calm down the activity of trigger points. However, manual therapists treat this problem quite differently, as will be explained later in the book (see pages 58–59).

ORTHOPEDIC CARE AND PHYSICAL THERAPY

Recent research has shown that:

- Nearly half of all patients who see their doctor because of backache are better within one week, whether or not they have treatment.

- After two weeks three out of four backaches will be better with or without treatment, whether medication, manipulation, or bed rest.

- Surveys of people who consulted their doctors for backache show that two months after the visit nine out of ten had no backache, again whether they had had some sort of treatment or no treatment at all.

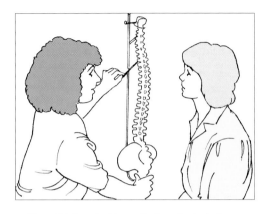

Above: *It is important to consider how often backaches recur and to evaluate whether appropriate treatment can prevent frequent recurrences, as well as reduce the severity of the symptoms in each patient.*

These results do not mean treatment is useless, because a great many of these people report that some form of attention provided ease and comfort. What we do know is that—apart from one person out of ten—the eventual result was the same, treatment or no treatment.

We also know that the one person in ten who still has a backache after two months probably has a severe problem, and it is important to know what can help this individual.

It is also important to consider how often backaches recur in many people, and to evaluate whether appropriate treatment can prevent frequent recurrences, as well as reduce the severity of symptoms.

Orthopedic and rheumatological care

Because doctors know most backaches get better on their own, they are most unlikely to refer patients with uncomplicated backache (that is backache which has no obvious pathology such as a disk prolapse or severe arthritis) to a specialist for treatment.

Patients who are referred to a specialist will usually have such severe discomfort and disability from their backache that an expert opinion is thought necessary. The urgency of such referrals is greater when there are obvious neurological signs and symptoms. Depending on what scans, tests, X-rays and so on have revealed, referral might be to a neurologist, to an orthopedic surgeon (in disk conditions), or to a rheumatologist (in cases of arthritis, for example).

For many years patients with severe backache resulting from disk dysfunction, especially where nerves were entrapped, were usually treated with traction or surgery.

Traction

In traction the patient is placed in a harness attached to a machine which gradually stretches the spine, either for a constant period or intermittently, pulling and then releasing the spine for a period of time in an attempt to reduce and relieve the pressure from the disk on sensitive local nerve and soft tissue structures. In cases of disk herniation traction is useful as part of the treatment protocol.

However, it is of little use for other forms of backache. The long-term results of traction are very poor, with a high rate of recurrence of symptoms before very long.

Surgery
Surgery of the spine is used when a disk herniation is so severe that normal functions like walking and standing are impossible without excruciating pain. Along with the use of spinal supports, this is discussed on pages 30–31

Drugs
Neurologists, rheumatologists, and orthopedic surgeons are likely to employ a variety of pharmaceutical drugs to help ease pain, inflammation, or active rheumatic disease. Among these are various steroid medications such as cortisone, which can provide amazing relief from severe symptoms but also produce a variety of severe side effects if taken long-term.

Physical therapy
Physical therapists employ a wide variety of machines, ranging from simple ultrasound and heat-emitting equipment to complex muscle-toning and relaxing gadgets, as well as exercise apparatus and hydrotherapy facilities. These are all designed to encourage the rehabilitation of muscles and areas which have become weak or dysfunctional.

Physical therapists are also increasingly using a large number of the manipulation and soft-tissue techniques employed by osteopaths and chiropractors, as well as a range of specialized exercise systems which have emerged from their own profession.

Exercise
Among the most successful exercise programs is the McKenzie system, which carefully examines a person's movement patterns and selects those which reduce pain as the basis for a sequence of organized, individualized exercises. Over time the regular performance of these progressive exercises, followed by retesting and prescribing new exercises, brings a profound improvement in many cases of both acute and chronic back pain—if the person with the problem is compliant and performs them regularly. This method, which selects exercises according to individual needs, achieves much better results than the "back schools" run in hospitals, where a standard set of exercises is taught to all those attending.

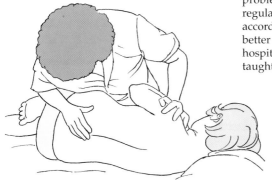

Left: Physical therapists are increasingly using the manipulation and soft-tissue techniques employed by osteopaths and chiropractors, as well as their own specialized exercise systems.

SURGERY

When back problems are accompanied by other symptoms such as referred pain down the leg (sciatica), muscle weakness, or loss of control of sphincters (bowel or bladder), and especially if some form of paralysis is present, mild or more severe, surgery may be an urgent option—but only if the cause is considered to be amenable to an operation which can remove pressure on the offending nerve root.

Operating on the spine is never a simple option, since research shows spinal surgery, such as compression of a nerve by a disk prolapse, fails far more often than it succeeds.

This is especially true if surgery is not accompanied by a range of rehabilitation and additional symptomatic treatment, including methods chosen from: traction; manipulation; reflex therapies (dealing with trigger points, for example); and spinal epidural injections.

Most importantly of all, rehabilitation exercises must be carefully chosen to meet the needs and demands of each individual.

Before deciding on surgery, if there is not a clear urgency as outlined in the previous paragraphs, many medical experts favor trying the more conservative methods. If no appreciable improvement is apparent after four to six weeks of whatever treatment combination is thought to be appropriate (traction, manipulation, medication, injections, or exercise) surgery should then be considered—but only if there is a real belief that the cause of the individual's pain and dysfunction can benefit from surgery.

A variety of surgical procedures are used, depending on the precise nature of the damage. Among the most common is the simple removal of the extruded pulp from the disk, taking away the cause of pressure on a nerve. In some cases the pulp can only be reached by first removing part of the bony structure of the spine; in such instances it may be necessary to fuse two vertebrae together after the removal of the pulp, using a graft of bone or some other method.

All these procedures involve major surgery and are commonly successful in removing at least some of the pain symptoms. The long-term outcome is more questionable because surgery often leaves the spine weaker and therefore vulnerable to future damage.

All such surgery should be accompanied by intensive rehabilitation programs with physical therapists. Usually, a comprehensive series of exercises are provided for the sufferer to do at home on a daily basis.

SPINAL FUSION

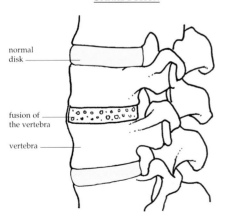

normal disk

fusion of the vertebra

vertebra

Left: A healthy disk is supple and acts as a shock-absorber. Once suppleness is lost and the bones of the spine fuse together (because of arthritis or medical intervention), stiffness results and the chance of injury increases.

SPINAL SUPPORTS

In some cases medical experts determine the spine requires immobilization by means of external support, either instead of, or after, surgery. In such cases corsets are prescribed to be worn when the person is upright. These do indeed provide support, but in doing so they encourage further progressive weakening of the muscles which should be performing the task naturally, sometimes making the person permanently dependent on a spinal support.

- There is certainly an argument for short-term use of elasticated support during acute episodes of backache, but anything more than a few days of wear can probably be avoided by appropriate use of carefully designed exercises and other home care (see Chapter 4 and previous pages).

- If an individual has extremely hypermobile (lax, loose) joints, supports may need to be worn long-term, and this may also be true of someone with recurrent back problems who has a prominent, sagging, abdomen.

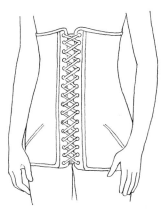

Above: Elasticated supports do, indeed, provide support, but in doing so they encourage further weakening of the muscles which should be performing the task.

This part of the recovery schedule is absolutely vital, as is the continued exercising which helps to strengthen the damaged area. Surgery itself produces major trauma to the functioning of the whole body, and it is the rehabilitation phase which is the key to the long-term success or failure of the operation.

Manipulation under anesthetic
Manipulation by osteopaths and chiropractors, and increasingly by physiotherapists, can be very gentle, as well as sometimes quite forceful, depending upon the area which requires attention and the particular requirements of the joint in question.

Orthopedic surgeons have adopted some of these methods, but usually employ them when the patient is fully anesthetized. The big advantage to this is that the patient cannot resist the manipulation, and the surgeon can then carefully position the spine, or area, to achieve the maximum benefit.

The disadvantage to the patient, apart from the side effects of a general anesthetic, is that they can offer no resistance to what is being done because their muscles are completely relaxed. This allows the possibility of severe force being applied to joints with the danger that they may be damaged because of this. While such an outcome occurs only rarely, it remains a risk.

CHAPTER THREE

PREVENTION

A rigid structure will break when stressed, while a flexible one will bend and absorb shocks and strains. Skyscrapers and bridges have built-in flexibility, and in much the same way the human spine is designed as a flexible structure and needs to be kept as supple as possible.

FLEXION EXERCISES: WHOLE BODY

The spine can flex (bend forward), extend (bend backward), and bend to each side, as well as rotating (twisting), when it is healthy and supple. As we age, and especially as we adapt to the multiple mechanical stresses and injuries of life, the muscles which support and move the spine, as well as other soft tissues such as the tendons and supporting fascia, and the joints themselves, can lose their ability to perform all these movements efficiently.

The exercises described on this and the following pages (pages 32–39) are designed to restore and maintain flexibility safely as far as possible.

NOTE 1 **If any of these exercises hurts while you are performing them, or leaves you in pain after its use, stop doing it.** Either the exercise is unsuitable for your back condition or you are performing it too energetically or repeating the exercise too often.

NOTE 2 Remember that the exercises in this chapter are "prevention" exercises, meant to be performed in a sequence so all the natural movements of the spine can benefit. They are *not* designed for treatment of back problems. Exercises for rehabilitation are described in Chapter 4.

Choose at least one of the following to perform at least once daily. (Ideally both exercises should be performed twice daily.)

Flexion exercise 1

- Time suggested: 4 minutes
- Repeat twice daily but not after a meal.

1) Sit on the floor with legs straight out in front of you, toes pointing toward the ceiling. Bend forward as far as is comfortable and grasp each leg with one hand. Let your head hang down.

2) Hold this position for 30 seconds. You should feel a stretch on the back of your legs and back. You should not feel any pain.

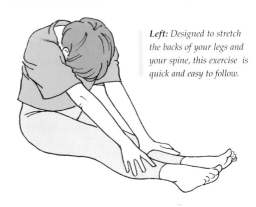

Left: Designed to stretch the backs of your legs and your spine, this exercise is quick and easy to follow.

3) As you release the fourth breath, ease yourself a little farther down your legs and grasp again. Stay here for about 30 seconds longer before slowly returning to an upright position.

4) Bend one leg and place the sole of your foot against the inside of the other knee, the bent knee as close to the floor as possible. Stretch forward down the straight leg and grasp it with both hands. Hold for 30 seconds as before and then, on an exhalation stretch farther down the leg and hold for 30 seconds longer.

5) Slowly return to an upright position and alter your legs so the one that was straight is now bent and the one that was bent is now straight. Repeat the sequence as described in step 4.

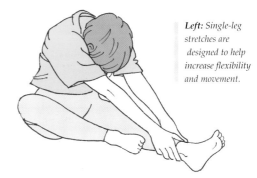

Left: Single-leg stretches are designed to help increase flexibility and movement.

6) Repeat steps 1-3 again.

Now move to a chair and perform flexion exercise 2.

Flexion exercise 2

- Suggested time: 2 to 3 minutes.
- Repeat twice daily but not after a meal.

1) Sit in a straight chair or on a stool with your feet about 8 inches apart. The palms of your hands should rest on your knees with fingertips facing inward toward each other. Lean forward so that the weight of your upper body is supported by your arms. Allow your elbows to bend outward and your head and chest forward. Make sure your head hangs forward. Hold the position where you feel the first signs of a stretch in your lower back.

2) Breathe in and out slowly and deeply three times. On exhalation, ease forward until you feel an increased, but not painful, stretch. Repeat the breathing. Repeat until you feel the stretch would be uncomfortable.

3) When and if you can fully bend in this position you should alter the exercise so that, sitting as described above, you are leaning forward, your head between your legs, with the backs of your hands resting on the floor. All other aspects of the exercise are the same, with you easing forward and down, bit by bit, staying in each new position for three to four breaths, before allowing a little more flexion to take place. Never let the degree of stretch be painful.

After performing either one or both of these flexion exercises, total time approximately six minutes, practice the two extension exercises which are described on pages 34-35.

Left: Stretch the spine gently using this simple exercise. As the flexibility builds the stretch will be easy.

EXTENSION EXERCISES: WHOLE BODY

Excessive extension (backward bending) of the spine is not desirable, and the "prevention" exercises outlined on these two pages are meant to be performed very gently, without any force or discomfort at all. Some people take the expression "no pain no gain" too literally. It is absolutely not true of spinal mobilization exercises such as these. The first exercise focuses on the whole spine, and the second one mainly on the upper back. **If you feel any pain, then stop doing the exercise.**

Choose at least one of the following exercises to perform a miminum of once daily. (In ideal circumstances both exercises should be performed twice daily.)

Extension exercise 1

- Time suggested: 2 minutes
- Repeat twice daily following flexion exercise.

1) Lie on your side (either side will do) on a carpeted floor with a small pillow to support your head and neck. Your legs should be together, one on top of the other.

2) Bend your knees as far as comfortably possible, bringing your heels toward your buttocks. Slowly move your upper legs (together)backward as far as you can, without pain, so your back is slightly arched. Your upper arm should rest along your side.

3) Take your head and shoulders backward to increase the backward bending of your spine. This should be done slowly and without pain— although you should be aware of a stretching sensation in the front of your body and some "crowding" in the middle of your back.

4) Hold this position for approximately three to four full breaths, and then hold your breath for about 15 seconds.

5) As you release this, try to ease first your legs and then your upper body into a little more extension. Hold this final position for about 30 seconds, breathing slowly and deeply all the while.

6) Bring yourself back to a straight side-lying position before turning on to your stomach for the next extension exercise.

Below: Curl your heels back toward your buttocks and then slowly move your upper legs back as far as you can. Keep your upper arm resting along your side.

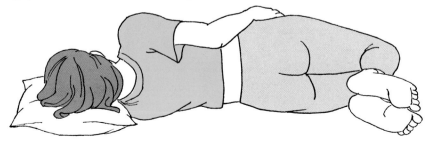

Extension exercise 2

- Time suggested: 2 minutes
- Five repetitions twice daily

Perform at least one of the flexion exercises as described on the previous pages, as well as the first extension exercise if possible, before performing this combined flexion and extension exercise.

1) On a carpeted floor, kneel on all fours, so that your weight rests on your knees and forearms, which should be positioned so your elbows are out to the side and the fingertips of each hand face each other. Your buttocks will be in the air and the rest of the back will slope downward toward your head.

2) To perform the exercise efficiently, bring your chin close to the floor, so your neck is bending backward and you are aware of a strained feeling in your upper back or base of your neck.

3) Imagine a small marble ball is on the carpet close to your hands, and you are going to roll this backward toward your knees—very slowly—with your chin, and then forward again in the same way.

4) Inhale and, as you slowly exhale, push the imaginary marble with your chin toward your knees, bringing your forehead close to the floor as you do so.

5) As you inhale return your head to the starting position and draw your shoulder blades together and hold for a second or two.

6) As you slowly exhale again take your chin to where you left "the marble"

near your knees, and slowly push it back to the starting position with your chin .

7) As you inhale lift your head, draw the shoulder blades together, hold for a second or two. As you exhale again repeat the whole sequence from the beginning.

8) Repeat the sequence five times altogether.

The breathing aspects of the exercise are crucial toits success, and you should take your time to ensure that you are moving into the "marble rolling" phase while breathing out, and that you are lifting your head backward and pulling your shoulder blades together as you breathe in. As you learn to do the exercise correctly, you will find it has a rhythmic quality. This exercise has a mobilizing effect on the area between the shoulder blades and upper spine, taking it through repeated flexion and extension motions.

You should expect to feel some discomfort during aspects of the exercise, but not pain. If you do feel pain, stop the exercise at once.

Below: Imagine a small marble ball is on the carpet close to your hands, and you are going to roll this backward and forward with your chin.

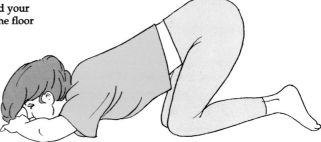

ROTATION EXERCISES: WHOLE BODY

These exercises should follow on from the flexion and extension exercises because they add the next important dimension to the self-mobilization sequence—rotation.

It is absolutely vital not to use any force when performing these exercises. Just take yourself to what is best described as an "easy barrier"—and never force yourself. You will slowly push the barrier back, as you become more supple, but these gains are achieved over a period of weeks or even months, not days. You will probably feel a little stiff and achy in newly stretched muscles the day after first performing the exercises. This will soon pass and does not require treatment of any sort.

Choose at least one of the following exercises to perform a minimum of once daily. (Ideally more than one of these exercises should be performed twice daily.)

Rotation exercise 1

- Time suggested: 4 minutes
- Repeat twice daily following flexion and extension exercises

1) Sit on a carpeted floor with legs outstretched. Bend your left leg and cross it over your right leg. Bring your right arm across your body and place your hand between your legs, on the floor by your right knee. This locks the knees in position.

2) Put your left hand behind your trunk and place it on the floor about 5 inches behind your buttocks with your fingers pointing backward. This twists your upper body to the left. Now turn your shoulders as far to the left as is comfortable without pain. Then turn your head to look over your left shoulder, as far as possible. Again make sure that you feel no pain, just stretch.

3) Stay in this position for five full, slow, breaths; then, as you breathe out, turn your shoulders and head a little farther to the left, to their new "restriction barriers."

4) Stay in this final position for an additional five full, slow, breaths.

5) Gently unwind yourself and repeat the whole exercise to the right, reversing all elements of the instructions. (In other words cross right leg over left, place left hand between knees, turn to the right and so on.)

Below: This exercise should be performed with care. Never overexert yourself during rotation exercises.

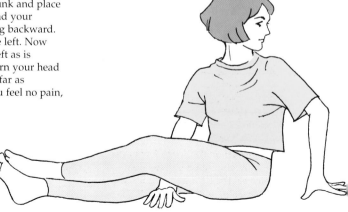

Rotation exercise 2

- Time suggested: 2 minutes
- Ideally repeat twice daily following at least one each of the flexion and extension exercises and ideally the previous rotation exercise.

1) Lie face upward on a carpeted floor with a small pillow or book under your head. Bend your knees so your feet, which should be together, are flat on the floor.

2) Keep your shoulders in contact with the floor during the exercise. This is helped by having your arms out to the side slightly, palms up.

4) Gently let your knees fall to the right as far as possible without pain—keeping your shoulders and your lower back in contact with the floor. You should feel a slight twisting sensation, but not a pain, in the muscles of the lower and middle parts of the back.

5) Hold this position while you breathe deeply and slowly for 30 seconds, as the weight of your legs "drags" on the rest of your body which is still, stretching a number of back muscles.

6) On an exhalation slowly bring your knees back to the midline. Then repeat the process in exactly the same manner, to the left side.

7) Repeat the exercise to both right and left once more, before straightening out and resting. Then follow the exercises on the next pages.

Below: Keep your shoulders in contact with the floor during the exercise. This is helped by having your arms out to the side slightly, palms upward.

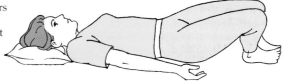

Rotation exercise 3

- Time suggested: 3 minutes
- Repeat twice daily instead of exercise 2.

1) Lie on the floor on your back with arms a little way out from the trunk, palms downward. Bend both knees and cross the left over the right and allow the weight of the left leg to take the left foot to the floor, dragging the right knee toward the floor. Your lower back will lift off the floor, but your shoulders should stay on the floor.

2) Lift your left foot from the floor a few inches and very gently pulse it toward the floor, rhythmically, ten times. You should feel a stretching sensation in the lower back.

If you feel any pain, stop immediately.

3) Reverse all positions, so the right leg crosses over the left and repeat the procedure as described.

Below: Bend both knees and cross the left over the right and allow the weight of the left leg to take the left foot to the floor, dragging the right knee toward the floor.

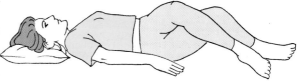

GENERAL MOBILITY: WHOLE BODY

The exercises described earlier help to improve and maintain mobility and suppleness in the muscles and structures which bend the spine backward, forward and rotate it. The exercises here farther increase spinal flexibility.

Perform one exercise daily. (Ideally more than one exercise should be performed twice daily.)

General mobility exercise 1

- Time suggested: 5 minutes
- Repeat whenever general stiffness is felt.

1) Stand with feet wide apart, but not stressfully so. Turn your left foot slightly to the left and the right foot facing in slightly—also to the left. Hold your arms out sideways at shoulder level, palms down.

2) Breathe in fully, and, as you exhale, bend sideways to the left, sliding your left hand down your left leg. Hold on to the leg with your hand when you have bent as far as you comfortably can. As you bend sideways take your right hand upward pointing toward the ceiling.

3) Turn your head to the right so you are looking upward at your right thumb. Make sure that you are not leaning forward or backward. Make sure your knees are straight and that your arms are fully stretched.

4) Stay in this position for a full minute, approximately six slow breaths in and out. After the sixth breath, as you exhale, stretch a little farther down your left leg with your left hand and hold this for a farther three breaths before slowly returning to the starting position.

5) Repeat the exercise on the opposite side (left hand toward ceiling, right hand down right leg and so on). A well-known yoga exercise, this is perfectly safe if you avoid force and bend only to the side, not forward or backward.

General mobility exercise 2

- Time suggested: 2 minutes
- Repeat twice daily

1) Lie flat on the floor with your arms by your side. Ease your legs to the right until you sense a degree of stretch in the left waist area.

2) Now ease your head and shoulders to the right as far as possible without strain, to create a side bend or "c" shape with your body.

3) Hold this position for three to four cycles of breathing. On the last inhalation, hold your breath for 10 to 15 seconds. As you exhale take your feet farther to the right and ease your right hand toward your feet, increasing the side bend. Hold this for another two breaths. Perform the same sequence to the left.

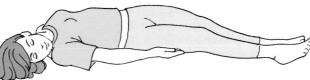

General mobility exercise 3

- Time suggested: 2 minutes
- Repeat twice daily if possible in a sequence which includes representative exercises from flexion, extension, and rotation

1) Lie flat on your back on a carpeted floor with both knees bent, feet comfortably apart and flat on the floor, and your hands locked behind your neck.

2) Bring the elbows together and raise your head off the floor by about 2 inches.

3) Repeatedly turn your trunk from one side to the other so one elbow touches the floor on each twist. Twist at least five times in each direction.

This movement will effectively stretch the muscles associated with the middle parts of your spine.

If the action of twisting hurts, stop the exercise immediately.

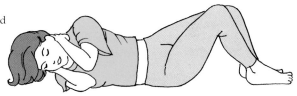

Below: Increase the general mobility of the spine with this gentle stretching exercise.

General mobility exercise 4

- Time suggested: 3 minutes
- Repeat whenever stiffness is felt in the upper back area.

This is also based on yoga principles. It is an ideal stretch of the areas between the shoulder blades and the front of the upper chest region.

1) Kneel on the floor and sit on your heels. If this is not possible, perform the exercise seated on an upright chair, or a stool, with your feet flat on the floor.

2) Ease your left hand behind your back and upward toward the right shoulder blade. At the same time take your right hand upward and back so that it can grasp your left hand, with fingers hooked together if possible.

3) Hold this stretch for four or five full, deep breaths. On an exhalation try to stretch just a little farther down your back with your right hand and up your back with your left hand. Stay in this position for a farther three to four breaths before slowly returning to the start position.

4) Repeat the entire sequence with the hands in the opposite positions.

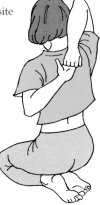

Right: This is a great exercise for stiffness in the upper areas of your back, between your shoulder blades, and the front of the upper chest region.

CHAPTER FOUR

REHABILITATION

Is your posture or breathing contributing to your backache? The exercises described in this chapter will help correct any problems, but you may require expert advice as well from a physical therapist, osteopath, chiropractor or other suitably qualified professional.

BREATHING RETRAINING

To check whether you need to do these exercises to correct your breathing, perform one or both of these tests.

- Sit on a chair in front of a mirror with your hands resting on your lap. Breathe deeply and watch your shoulders. Do they rise toward your ears? If they do, you are over using the upper fixator muscles of the neck and shoulders (see pages 24–25)

- Sit on a chair in front of a mirror and place one hand flat on your stomach area, just below your ribs and above your navel. Place the other hand flat on your upper chest. Take a deep breath and watch your hands. If the upper hand moves first, or the most, and especially if it moves upward toward your throat, the test is positive.

If in the first test your shoulders rose, or if the second test was positive—and especially if you also have back problems—your breathing pattern is probably contributing to any backache you suffer. The exercises described below will assist in normalizing the process.

To start to retrain breathing and to help reduce any tendency toward hyperventilation and consequent stress on your back, you should perform the following exercises regularly, preferably every day.

Breathing exercise 1

1) Get comfortable, ideally seated/reclining, with both hands resting on the stomach just below your ribs. Now exhale fully and slowly through your partially open mouth, lips barely separated. This out breath should be controlled and unhurried. Imagine a candle flame is about 7 inches from your mouth and exhale in such a way as to blow a stream of air gently toward it without blowing it out. As you exhale in this way count silently to establish the length of the out breath. An effective method for counting one second at a time is to think to yourself "one hundred, two hundred, three hundred and so on." Each count then lasts about one second.

2) When you have exhaled fully, without causing any feeling of strain, allow the inhalation which follows to be full, free, and uncontrolled. The complete exhalation which preceded the inhalation will have created a "coiled spring" which you do not have to control in order to inhale. Once again count to yourself to establish how long your in-breath lasts. You need to count because the timing of

the inhalation and exhalation phases of breathing is an important feature of this exercise.

3) Without pausing to hold your breath in, exhale again in the same way as described, through the mouth (again you count to yourself at the same speed). Repeat the inhalation/exhalation cycles 15 to 20 times.

5) Your hands should become aware of a slight "push forward" as you inhale, and a flattening of the stomach as you exhale, but do not try to control these movements. They indicate your diaphragm is beginning to work correctly.

6) The objective of this exercise is that in time you should achieve an inhalation phase which lasts for two to three seconds while the exhalation phase lasts from six to eight seconds—without any strain at all. This is unlikely at first and all you should try to make sure happens is that exhaling takes longer than inhaling.

7) Most important, the exhalation should be slow and continuous. It is no use breathing the air out in two seconds and then simply waiting until the count reaches 6, 7, or 8 before inhaling again.

8) By the time you have completed 15 or so cycles, your awareness of pain should have lessened and any sense of anxiety which may underlie your pain also should be much reduced.

9) Repeat this exercise at least every morning and ideally several times daily.

Below: Learning to breath correctly is an important part of the rehabilitation process.

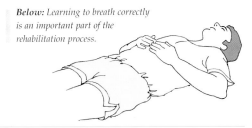

Breathing exercise 2

1) Sit in a chair which has arms, and rest your arms on the chair. As you practice deep breathing make sure your elbows are pressed firmly downward toward the floor, against the arms of the chair, all the time.

3) As you practice deep breathing (to the timing described in the previous exercise), try to observe whether or not—without making any particular effort to make it happen—your abdomen moves forward at the start of inhalation and flattens on exhalation. While pressing down with the elbows it is impossible to use the neck/shoulder muscles; so you are obliged to use correct breathing muscles.

4) Do this exercise a number of times each day if possible, for about five cycles of breathing each time—until you can sit in front of a mirror and inhale without shoulders lifting.

In addition to these exercises you should perform the muscle stretches outlined on pages 49–51 and mobility exercise 3 on page 39.

Left: Without trying to influence your abdomen, observe whether it moves forward on inhalation and flattens on exhalation.

POSITIONAL RELEASE RULES

When we feel pain, the area which is troubled will usually have some degree of local muscle tension, even spasm. There is probably a degree of local circulatory deficiency as well, with not enough oxygen getting to the troubled area and not enough of the normal waste products being removed from the troubled area.

Massage and stretching methods can often help reduce the pain in these situations, even if only temporarily. However, massage is not always available, or may be impractical if the region is out of reach and you are on your own. If the back pain problem is very severe, stretching may also be too uncomfortable to try—although safe and very gentle ways of stretching are explained on pages 44–45.

There is another way of easing tense, tight muscles, and improving local circulation. It is called "positional release technique" (PRT).

It has been found in osteopathic medicine that almost all painful conditions relate in some way to areas which have been strained or stressed in some way—either quickly in a sudden accident or incident, or gradually over time because of bad habits of use, posture and so on.

PRT experiment

1) Sit in a chair and press into your neck just behind your jaw, directly below your ear lobe. Most of us have painful muscles here. Press just hard enough to hurt a little, and grade this pain for yourself as a "10" (where " 0" is no pain).

2) While still pressing the point, slowly bend your neck forward so that your chin moves toward your chest. Keep deciding what the "score" is in the painful point.

3) As soon as you feel the pain ease, start turning your head in the direction of the pain, until the pain drops again. By "fine tuning" the position of your head, you should be able to get the score close to"0."

4) When you find that position, you have taken the pain to its position of "ease." Stay in that position (but do not press on the point) for about half a minute and then sit up. You should find the painful area is less sensitive—and the area will have been flushed with fresh oxygenated blood.

5) If this was a real painful area, not an "experimental" one, the pain would ease over the next day or two.

You can try this technique on any pain point anywhere on the body. It may not cure the problem (although sometimes it will), but it offers some relief.

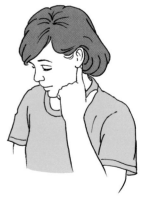

Above: Finding the pain point and taking it to its position of "ease" will help the problem.

When these "strains"—whether they are acute or chronic—develop, some tissues (muscles, fascia, ligaments, tendons, nerve fibers and so on) are unduly stretched and others become unnaturally shortened.

It is not surprising pain will develop out of such a pattern, or that these tissues will be more likely to become painful when asked to do something out of the ordinary, such as lifting or stretching. They will have lost their normal elasticity, at least in part, in the shortened structures. It is, therefore, not uncommon for recent strains of the back or elsewhere to occur in tissues which are already chronically stressed in some way. Only by applying the exercises in this book will the underlying problem be solved and the muscles returned to their normal states.

It has been found in PRT that gently easing the tissues which are short into a position in which they are made even shorter, a degree of comfort or "ease" is achieved which can help to remove pain from the area.

But how are we to know which way to move tissues which are very painful and tense?

There are some very simple rules which we can apply ourselves using the simple experiment shown on page 42.

SELF APPLICATION OF PRT

THE RULES FOR SELF APPLICATION OF PRT ARE -

- Locate a painful point and press hard enough to score "10."

- If the point is on the front of the body bend forward to ease it. The farther from the midline of your body the more you should ease yourself to that side.

- If the point is on the back of the body ease backward and away from the side of the pain. Then "fine tune" to achieve ease.

- Hold the position of ease for not less than 30 seconds and very slowly return to the neutral starting position.

- No pain should be produced elsewhere when finding the position of ease.

- Do not treat more than five pain-points on any one day.

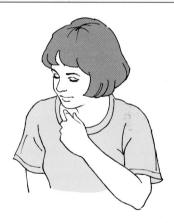

Above: Once in the position of "ease," no pain should be produced elsewhere in the body.

- Expect improvement in function—ease of movement—fairly soon (minutes) after such self treatment: reduction in pain may take a day or so.

MUSCLE ENERGY TECHNIQUES

When a muscle has been contracted, without any movement being allowed, for around ten seconds something quite remarkable occurs to it and to its antagonist(s)—the muscle or muscles which perform the opposite action to the muscle being contracted.

They will all be far more relaxed than they were before the contraction, and so the muscle which has been contracted and its antagonist(s) can be stretched much more easily than previously. We will be using muscle energy methods such as this to prepare a muscle for stretching if it is found to be shorter and tighter than it ought to be, and so inhibiting, weakening, its antagonist.

A muscle that is short and tight is not necessarily weak, though it might be. What is certain is that its antagonist will be weaker than it should be, and that it will be unable to regain strength until the cause of the weakness is removed. This cause is often the extra tightness or shortness we are about to discover how to stretch.

The sort of contraction we will use is known as an isometric (iso = equal, metric = measure) contraction. This occurs when you push against an immovable object—your muscles are working, they are contracting, but they are not moving anything.

Obviously it is possible to push or pull against a heavy object with all your strength, but in this sort of exercise we are looking for light contractions only—often described as "no more than a quarter of your available strength."

The use of isometric muscle contractions in this way is known in osteopathic and physical medicine as "muscle energy technique."

Practitioners and therapists use these techniques widely, but what is described in this book are a number of self-applied muscle energy techniques (MET).

A small experiment will help you to understand just how we can use the benefits of MET.

MET exercise

1) Sit close to a table with your elbows on the table and rest your hands on each side of your face. Turn your head as far as you can comfortably turn it in one direction, say to the right, letting your hands move with your face, until you reach your limit of rotation.

2) Now use your left hand to resist your attempt to turn your head back toward the left, using no more than a quarter of your strength. Start the turn slowly, building up force which is matched by your left hand. Hold this push—with no movement at all taking place—for seven to ten seconds, and then slowly stop your effort to turn your head left. Now ease your head round to the right. You should find you can turn a good deal farther than the first time you tried the contraction. You have been using MET to achieve post-isometric relaxation.

3) Your hands should still be each side of your face. Now use your right hand to resist your attempt to turn even farther to the right, starting slowly, and maintaining the turn and the resistance for a full seven to ten seconds.

4) When your effort slowly stops, see if you can now go even farther to the right than after your first two efforts. You have been using MET to achieve reciprocal inhibition.

ISOMETRIC TECHNIQUES

RECIPROCAL INHIBITION (RI)

POST-ISOMETRIC RELAXATION (PIR)

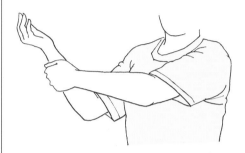

Above: Resisting an attempt to move the arm with isometric contractions is a way of using the muscle energy technique.

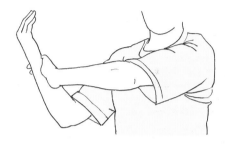

Above: Stopping the arm bending is another way of using the muscle energy technique.

You have been using MET in its two modes, using the muscles which need releasing and then using antagonists.

Both methods work to release tightness for about 20 seconds and both will allow you the chance to stretch the tight muscles. The MET contractions work by stimulating particular nerve reflexes, and so are working with normal body functions to achieve a release of undesirable excessive tightness.

On the following pages when MET is described we will use only the first method (post-isometric relaxation), contracting the muscle which needs to be released.

Sometimes you will use an object such as stool or a step, and sometimes gravity as the force against which you will be contracting the muscle in question. Sometimes you will use your own hand contact(s), just as you did with your neck in the exercise on the previous page.

Whichever you use the effect will be the same, a more relaxed muscle which can then be more easily stretched.

In many of the exercises described on pages 32-39 and those which will be outlined on pages 52-57 it is possible to utilize muscle energy techniques (MET) by contracting whatever parts of the body are being stretched for a few seconds just before you move to a new, more stretched position.

In fact, most yoga stretches employ MET without, perhaps, being aware of its mechanisms. This may be one of the reasons yoga is such an effective system of exercise and relaxation.

HAMSTRINGS AND PSOAS MUSCLES

The two muscles discussed on these pages are important for the back because of their intimate relationship with the pelvis (hamstrings) and the spine itself (psoas). To know whether or not they require stretching, you can perform simple self-assessment tests.

Neither of these very large structures can "release" and normalize in just one session of stretching, so repetitions are required on a daily basis for some weeks before short and tight muscles become supple again and reach something like their normal length.

The advice offered on these pages is not meant to replace professional attention, but is suggested as a means of helping yourself whatever else is being done for your back problem. None of these methods should hurt (apart from some tenderness and stiffness the day after you first perform the stretches).

If you feel pain, stop the exercise immediately.

Hamstring self-assessment test
The hamstrings are the main muscles of the back of the leg and are active every time you take a step. They anchor on to the bone on which you sit, the ischium, and have a major influence on the function of the pelvis and the lower back.

- Sit on the floor with legs out straight. Bend slowly forward with hands outstretched toward the toes. If you find that you cannot reach your toes without a strong stretching sensation in the back of the thighs, your hamstring muscles are probably short. There can be other reasons for not reaching your toes, but tight hamstrings are the most likely.

- Exercise 1 on page 32 will effectively stretch these muscles, and should be performed daily if not painful to the back.

Hamstring MET self-treatment: Method 1

1) Stand in front of a chair or box, 18-24 inches high. Place the leg to be stretched half a pace behind you and the other with the foot flat on the surface of the chair or box so your toes and the ball of your foot, but not your heel, are resting on it.

2) Rest your hands on your bent knee, and, keeping a straight back all the time, lean forward until you feel a slight pull on the back of your straight leg.

3) Now, using about 20 percent of your strength, push your straight knee backward,

contracting the muscles at the back of the leg, for about ten seconds.

4) When you have finished this push ease yourself farther forward stretching the muscles behind the leg.

5) Repeat this exercise three times.

Left: Rest your hands on your bent knee, and, keeping a straight back all the time, lean forward until you feel a slight pull along the back of your straight leg.

Hamstring MET self-treatment: Method 2

1) Stand with one foot on a stool or chair back, leg straight, heel resting on the surface. Your hands should be resting on your leg just below the knee.

2) Now lean forward until you feel a slight stretch at the back of the leg on the stool. Push downward with that leg into the stool with your heel, using about 20 percent of your strength (too much effort can trigger a cramp so do not try too hard!) for ten seconds.

3) After you have stopped pushing down, ease yourself farther forward to increase the stretch. Repeat four times altogether.

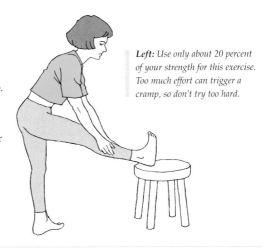

Left: Use only about 20 percent of your strength for this exercise. Too much effort can trigger a cramp, so don't try too hard.

Psoas self-assessment test

Psoas is a very important muscle which runs from your hip, over the front of the pelvis, through your abdomen, to anchor on to the front of your spine. One of its main roles is to bend your hip, as when walking.

- Lie on your back on the floor with your knees bent, feet flat on the floor and slightly apart, and arms folded on to your chest.

- Raise your head and then your shoulders and, if you can, your shoulder blades from the floor. If you can do this without your feet (either or both) leaving the floor, or feeling as though they want to, your psoas muscles are not short. If they are, do the exercise here.

Right: The exercise here is designed to help stretch your psoas muscles if they are short.

Psoas MET self-treatment

1) Stand on the floor at the end of your bed and then sit down on the very edge. Bring the knee of the side you are not treating (both may need stretching but you have to do these one at a time) up to your chest and hold it firmly there with both hands.

2) Roll backward on to the bed and allow the leg on the side you are treating to hang freely. Raise the knee of that leg into the air by about 4 inches and hold it there for ten seconds.

3) Slowly release and let the leg hang free again, with gravity providing the stretch, for 20 seconds longer. Repeat four times altogether and then stretch the other side in the same way. Do this daily until the test no longer indicates the psoas is short.

QUADRATUS LUMBORUM AND TENSOR FASCIA LATA MUSCLES

Quadratus self-assessment test

Quadratus lumborum (QL) is an important muscle which bends your spine sideways. It runs from the crest of your pelvis to the spine at around waist level. Just like psoas, described earlier, QL has fibers which merge with your diaphragm. This means that if either of these muscles is short, it will pull and drag on this part of your breathing apparatus, and can contribute to some of the difficulties described on pages 24 –25. If you are trying to normalize breathing function by means of the exercises on pages 40–41, it makes sense to stretch any muscles which might be add to the problem.

None of these methods should hurt (apart from some tenderness and stiffness the day after you first perform the stretches).

Quadratus MET self-treatment

1) Stand as in the test position and bend sideways away from the side to be treated, making sure you do not also bend forward or backward at all. When you have reached as far as you can, running your hand down the side of your leg, inhale and come back up about two inches. Stay in this position for ten seconds.

2) On exhaling, release your effort and slide your hand down the leg a little farther than you could before. Stay in that stretch position for another ten seconds.

3) Repeat until you are not gaining any more length. Then treat the other side if necessary. Repeat daily until you can reach a good two inches past your knee without effort.

If pain is felt you should stop the exercise immediately.

- Stand with your legs shoulder-width apart and bend slowly to one side as far as you can without pain, and without lifting the foot on the side from which you are bending. See how far your fingertips reach on the leg toward which you are bending. It should be several inches past the knee.

- Now perform the same bend on the other side. The length here should also be several inches past the knee. If you cannot reach as far to the left as you can to the right, then QL on the right is probably shortened, so preventing easy bending on that side. If you cannot reach past your knee on either side then both QLs are short and need stretching.

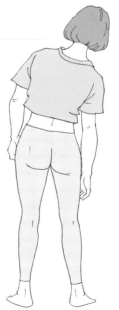

Left: Gently stretching the quadratus lumborum will not only help the structure of the body, but will also help your breathing.

Tensor fascia lata self-assessment test

Tensor fascia lata (TFL) is the muscle/fascia structure which runs down the side of your leg, from above your hip joint to below your knee. It helps to lift your leg sideways, and is important to the mechanics of the back because it anchors to your pelvis.

If it is short it can change the way the pelvis moves, causing stress in the back. Shortness of TFL can also cause knee problems.

● Lie on your side so you are perfectly square to the surface, not rolling forward or backward at all. Your lower leg should be bent at the knee and hip to provide stability, preventing your trunk from rolling forward.

● Rest your head on your bent lower arm. Make sure that your upper leg lies in a straight line with your trunk. Slowly raise it sideways toward the ceiling. Does it seem to come forward at all?

● If it does, the TFL is short and needs stretching. If you cannot see for yourself whether the leg drifts forward on being raised, ask someone else to give you an opinion. It should stay exactly in line with the trunk.

TFL MET self-treatment

1) Lie on your side on a bed with your hips very close to the end.

2) Draw the lower leg toward your chest while allowing the upper one to hang over the edge.

3) Introduce an isometric contraction, against gravity, by raising the upper leg toward the ceiling a few inches.

4) Hold this position for at least ten seconds before slowly releasing the leg so gravity can introduce a stretch to the shortened muscle.

5) Let the leg hang down like this for a good 20 seconds.

6) Repeat the contraction and stretch at least three more times.

This is a very "tough" band of muscle and fascia and it can take several months to stretch it effectively. However, it is well worth the effort if it is thought to be short.

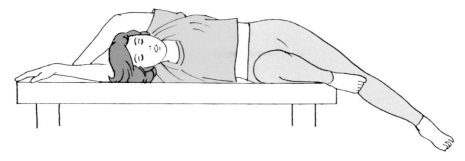

Below: Introducing an isometric contraction against gravity helps release the shortness in the TFL muscle.

UPPER TRAPEZIUS AND LEVATOR SCAPULAR MUSCLES

Both the upper trapezius and the levator scapular muscles are "accessory breathing muscles," which means they work when needed in the breathing process, but they do not work all the time.

If your breathing patterns are disturbed, such as in conditions like asthma or when stressed with hyperventilation (see pages 24–25 and pages 40–41), these muscles become stressed and, because they are postural muscles (see pages 14–15), they shorten.

In many cases of upper-back problems, these important muscles will need stretching for the underlying conditions to be remedied.

Upper trapezius MET self-treatment

1) Lie on your back on the floor, with a pillow under your head. If treating the left upper trapezius, lift your left buttock, stretch your left arm down and lie on it. Take your right hand up over your head and stretch your head and neck sideways to the right as far as is comfortable.

2) With your head and arm in this position, gently shrug the left shoulder and at the same time try to take your left ear toward the left shoulder, while resisting this with your right hand.

3) Keep these contractions going for approximately ten seconds, using no more than 20 percent of your strength.

Right: The upper trapezius muscles are "accessory breathing muscles" and will become shortened if breathing patterns are disturbed. This exercise helps to stretch them again.

Upper trapezius self-assessment test

Upper trapezius runs from the shoulder to the neck and commonly houses a number of painful trigger points (pages 58–59) which refer pain to the neck, and head as well as the upper back.

- Sit on a chair and place your left hand on the muscle which lies between your right shoulder and your neck. Curve your fingers backward so that they can feel movement in the muscle during the test. Take your right arm backward as you would when swinging your arms.

- Is there any contraction of muscle under your fingers? There should not be and if there is upper trapezius is overworking, and therefore shortened and in need of stretching.

4) On releasing, lift your left buttock and stretch the left arm farther down before lying on it again.

5) At the same time ease your head and neck farther to the right in a painless stretch. Hold this for ten seconds. Repeat twice more before treating the other side, if needed.

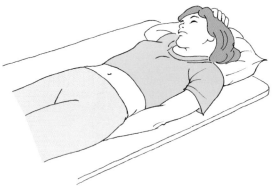

Levator scapula self-assessment test

Levator scapula is a muscle which lifts the shoulder blade, as well as providing stability so any arm movement is easy (the upper arm has a joint with the shoulder blade at the shoulder joint).

When it is short, levator scapula can create problems for the upper back, neck and shoulder. In most adults, levator scapula has active trigger points (see pages 58-59) which refer pain into the upper and middle back as well as the shoulder and neck. Try this self-assessment test to see if your levator scapula is short and requires treatment to lengthen it.

- Sit in front of a mirror and hold your arm out sideways. Bend the elbow so that your hand points forward, and hold your arm just below the level of the shoulder. Slowly raise your elbow, allowing your hand to hang down a little.

- Observe what happens between your neck and shoulder joint. Do the muscles in this area stay "flat" or do they "bunch"?

- If they do bunch, then levator scapula is shortened (and usually the upper trapezius as well) and both need stretching.

Levator scapula MET self-treatment

1) The treatment position for levator scapula is almost identical to that of upper trapezius. The difference is that instead of simply sidebending the flexed neck (which just as in upper trapezius should be bent forward and supported on a pillow), the neck is both side bent and fully rotated, turned away from the side being treated. If you are treating left levator, flex your neck, sidebend it to the right and turn it to the right. Use your right hand to hold it this position.

2) Once again you should anchor the arm on the side to be treated underneath your buttock. In this position introduce two isometric contractions. The first involves pushing your head back toward its original position against the resistance of your own hand (20 percent strength only). The other—at the same time—involves shrugging the left shoulder (in this example) against the resistance of the weight of your body which is lying on it.

3) Hold the contractions for about ten seconds. On release lift your buttock and stretch farther down and lie on the arm again, while at the same time painlessly increasing the amount of flexion, sidebending, and rotation of the neck with your right hand. Hold the stretch for about ten seconds before treating twice more. Perform exactly the same sequence on the other side if needed.

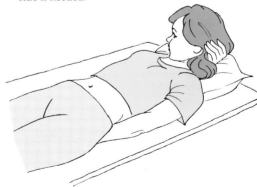

Right: The treatment position for the levator scapula muscle is almost identical to that of upper trapezius, except that the flexed neck is bent forward and fully rotated.

REHABILITATION CHAIR EXERCISES

These chair-based exercises are intended to be used when you already have or have recently had back pain. You should use them only if they offer appreciable relief from current symptoms.

Chair exercise to improve spinal flexion

1) Sit in an upright chair, feet about 8 inches apart. Twist slightly to the right and bend forward as far as comfortably possible so your left arm hangs between your legs. Make sure your neck is free so your head hangs down. You should feel a stretching sensation between your shoulders and in your lower back.

2) Stay in this position for about 30 seconds (approximately four slow, deep breaths). On an exhalation ease your left hand toward your right foot a little more and stay in this position for 30 seconds longer.

3) On an exhalation, stop the left-hand stretch and ease your right hand toward the floor just to the right of your right foot. Hold this position for another 30 seconds.

4) Slowly sit up again and turn a little to your left. Bend forward so your right arm hangs between your legs. Make sure your neck is free so your head hangs down. Once again you should feel a stretching sensation between your shoulders and in your lower back.

Right: If your back is already painful, you should always consult a suitably qualified health care professional before doing any of the exercises given here.

Do not do the exercises if they cause you pain.
If you have a problem which requires regular treatment, whether this is manual or medication, or if there is any suggestion you may have a disk condition, consult a suitably qualified health-care professional before doing any of the exercises given here.

5) Stay in this position for about 30 seconds. On an exhalation ease your right hand toward your left foot and stay in this position for another 30 seconds. On an exhalation stop this stretch with your right hand. Begin to stretch your left hand to the floor just to the left of your left foot and hold this position for another 30 seconds. Sit up slowly and rest for a minute before resuming normal activities or doing the next exercise.

Exercise 2 on pages 32–33 is another safe chair-based exercise to encourage general spinal flexion mobility during rehabilitation.

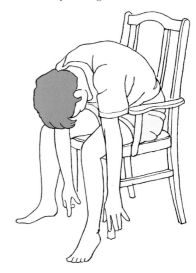

Chair exercise to improve upper-back mobility

1) Sit in an upright chair and stretch your arms out sideways with fingers widely spread. Rotate your arms at the shoulder so your left thumb points upward and your right thumb points downward.

2) Turn your head fully toward the right (the side on which the thumb is down). Hold this position for a count of five. Rotate your arms so that your left thumb is down and your right thumb points upward. As you do this turn your head toward the left—the thumb down side.

Right: Synchronize the movements so that your head turns and your arms rotate as you inhale deeply, and hold the position as you exhale.

3) Begin to synchronize these alternations so you perform the head turn and the arm rotation on a deep inhalation, holding the position during the slow exhalation, and repeating the changes on the next inhalation. Repeat the cycle of head turn and arm rotation for approximately 15 repetitions, to mobilize the area between your shoulder blades.

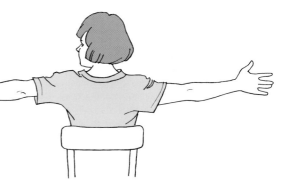

Chair exercise to encourage spinal mobility in all directions

1) Sit in an upright chair and lean sideways so your right hand grasps the back right leg of the chair. On an exhalation slowly slide your hand down the leg as far as is comfortable, and hold this position, partly supporting yourself with your hand. Stay in this position for two or three breaths before sitting up on an exhalation.

2) Now ease yourself forward and grasp the front right chair leg with your right hand, and repeat the exercise as described above. Follow this by holding on to the left front leg and finally the left back leg with your left hand and repeating all the elements as described. Make two or three "circuits" of the chair in this way to slowly increase your range of movement.

Chair exercise to improve rotation flexibility

1) Sit facing the back of an upright chair with feet flat on the floor. Interlock your fingers in front of you (palms upward) and make sure that your elbows are pointing out sideways fully.

2) Now inhale. As you exhale turn your head and your trunk to one side leading with your elbows, making suring that your feet stay flat and you stay firmly seated—do not lift one side of your buttocks as you turn. While in the turned position breathe in deeply again. As you exhale turn fully to the other side, and stay there while you inhale fully.

3) Repeat the turns from side to side as you exhale for a total of ten cycles. This exercise will help to mobilize the middle and lower back, as well as the ribs.

REHABILITATION PRONE EXERCISES

There are a number of exercises which can be safely performed in the face-down position, or on all-fours, during the rehabilitation phase of a back problem—if, that is, they produce no pain during their performance.

The exercises described on these pages are almost always well tolerated and are safe for most back problems, but you should avoid them if you have an active disk condition or a spondylolisthesis (a condition in which the last vertebra of the spine "slips" forward of its contact with the sacrum), a situation which shows up very easily on an X-ray or scan.

Prone rehabilitation exercise 1

1) This is especially useful for mobilizing the area just above the waist. Kneel all fours so that your weight is on your knees and your hands. Your hands should be placed directly below your shoulders, facing forward. As you inhale, round your back into an arch, pushing upward toward the ceiling with your spine and at the same time dropping your head downward between your arms. Imagine your navel is being pulled upward to touch the spine, so you actually retract and pull in your abdomen during the arching of the back.

2) Hold this position and your breath for a slow count of ten, then slowly exhale. As you do so lower your arched spine toward the floor and bring your head upward so you are looking straight ahead. Hold this position and breathe out for a count of five, before inhaling slowly again and arching your back at the same time—repeating the first phase of the exercise. Perform all movements very slowly and try to achieve a synchronization with the breathing cycle as described. Repeat five times (arch upward five times and downward five times), finishing with an upward arch.

3) To achieve a more focused mobilization of the upper back, perform exactly the same sequence with your weight supported on your knees and elbows (rather than hands as in 1). Your elbows should rest on the floor just below your ears, forearms, beside each other below your head.

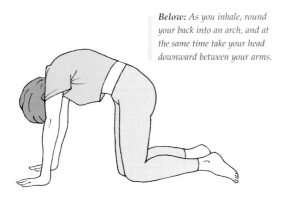

Below: As you inhale, round your back into an arch, and at the same time take your head downward between your arms.

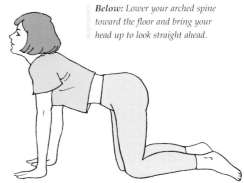

Below: Lower your arched spine toward the floor and bring your head up to look straight ahead.

Prone rehabilitation exercise 2

1) Lie flat on your stomach with your arms lying by your sides. Inhale, raise one leg into the air, and hold for a count of five. As you slowly exhale, lower the leg to the floor and rest for one inhalation/exhalation cycle.

2) On the next inhalation raise the other leg and hold for a count of five before lowering on the exhalation and resting for one cycle. On the next inhalation raise both legs slightly from the floor and hold for five seconds, if possible, before lowering on an exhalation and resting for one cycle. If you have achieved these leg raises without discomfort, proceed to the next phase.

3) This time, on an inhalation, raise one leg as well as your head and shoulders and hold for a count of five, before lowering and resting as before for a cycle of inhalation and exhalation.

4) Next raise the other leg as well as your head and shoulders, hold for five seconds, then lower and rest. Next raise both legs and your head and shoulders, hold for five seconds, lower and rest.

5) Repeat the leg, head, and shoulder raising five times with each leg as well as with both legs together, if possible. If any of this is too difficult at first, just perform the leg lifts without the head and shoulder raising, until that movement becomes possible.

6) The exercise will effectively tone many of the spinal muscles which may have become weakened during a period of inactivity. If any aspect of the exercise actually hurts leave it out, but perform those aspects of the exercise which are not uncomfortable. With practice you may be able to incorporate more and more of the sequence.

Prone rehabilitation exercise 3

1) Lie face down, legs out straight, stomach on the floor but head and shoulders off the floor, supporting yourself on your elbows, hands pointing forward—in a sphinx position.

Below: Every tenth breath, breathe in slowly and very slightly straighten your arms so that you feel a little stretch in the small of your back.

2) Every tenth breath or so, breathe in slowly and very slightly straighten the arms so you feel a little stretch in the small of your back.

3) Hold this for one or two cycles of breathing before resting back on to your elbows and remain in this position for up to five minutes, repeating the extension (back-bending) sequence every tenth breath.

4) This exercise effectively encourages flexibility in backward bending. Do not do it if it hurts.

Avoid prone rehabilitation exercises if you have a disk problem or spondylolisthesis.

REHABILITATION SUPINE EXERCISES

In order for the back to be stable and strong some of the abdominal muscles must receive attention. Like the guy ropes of a tent pole, they should be neither slack nor excessively tight, or imbalances will occur and the strain from these will probably affect the spine.

The exercises on these pages are designed to help normalize the weak abdominal muscles, as well as to stretch the low back from this position (exercises 1 and 2). This can farther strengthen the abdominal muscles by taking away weakening influences as discussed on pages 20-21.

Supine rehabilitation exercise for lower back and pelvic muscles

1) Lie on the floor on your back with a pillow under your head. Keep your lower back flat to the floor throughout the exercise. As you exhale draw your right hip toward the shoulder—as though you were "shrugging it." At the same time stretch your left leg away from you (push the heel away not the pointed toe), trying to make it longer.

2) Hold this for a few seconds before inhaling again and relaxing both efforts. Repeat in the same way on the other side, drawing the left leg up and pushing the right leg away. Repeat the sequence five times altogether.

3) This exercise stretches the muscles just above the pelvis and is very useful following a period of inactivity due to back problems.

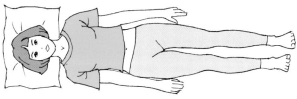

Supine rehabilitation exercise for abdominal muscles and pelvis

1) Lie on your back on a carpeted floor, without a pillow, knees bent, and arms folded over your abdomen. As you inhale and hold your breath, do all the following at the same time.

● Pull your abdomen in ("as if you were trying to staple your navel to your spine")

● Tilt the pelvis forward by flattening your back to the floor

● Squeeze your buttocks tightly together

● Lift your hips toward the ceiling.

2) Hold this combined contraction for a slow count of five before exhaling and relaxing onto the floor for a another cycle of breathing. Repeat five to ten times.

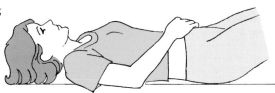

Supine rehabilitation exercise to tone abdominal muscles

1) Lie on the floor with your knees bent and arms folded across your chest. Push your lower back toward the floor and tighten your buttock muscles.

2) As you inhale, raise your head, neck, and, if possible, your shoulders from the floor—even if it is only a little way. Hold this for five seconds.

3) As you exhale, relax all tight muscles and lie on the floor for a full cycle of relaxed breathing before repeating.

Below: As you inhale raise your head, neck, and, if possible, your shoulders from the floor—even if it is only a little way.

4) Repeat this up to ten times to strengthen the abdominal muscles.

5) When you can do this relatively easily, add this simple variation. As you lift yourself from the floor, ease your right elbow toward your left knee—hold as above and then relax. The next lift should take the left elbow toward the right knee. This strengthens the oblique abdominal muscles.

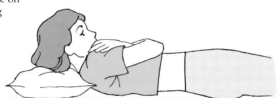

Supine rehabilitation exercise for lower back and abdominals

1) Lie on your back on a carpeted floor, with a small pillow under your head. Bend one knee and hip and hold the knee with both your hands.

2) Inhale deeply and, as you exhale, draw the knee to the shoulder on the same side, as far as is comfortably possible. Repeat this two more times.

3) Rest that leg on the floor and perform the same sequence with the other leg. Replace the second leg on the floor. Now bend both legs at both the knee and hip and clasp one knee with each hand.

3) Have your knees comfortably apart (shoulder-width ideally) and draw your knees toward your shoulders—not your chest.

4) When you feel a slight stretch in the lower back, inhale deeply.

5) Hold the breath and the position for ten seconds, before slowly releasing the breath and at the same time easing your knees a little closer toward your shoulders.

6) Repeat the sequence of inhalation and held breath followed by the easing of the knees closer to the shoulders an additional four times (five times in all).

7) After the fifth stretch to the shoulders, stay in the final position for about half a minute while breathing deeply and slowly.

This exercise effectively stretches many of the lower and middle muscles of the back. It is particularly useful if any of the flexion exercise sequences (pages 32-33) are uncomfortable to perform.

ACUPRESSURE AND TRIGGER POINT TREATMENT

A trigger point is an area of muscle which has become stressed through injury, overuse, or poor posture, and in which the nerves have become sensitive and very easily irritated. A trigger point hurts locally and also causes pain at a distance from itself, in a "target area."

Acupressure is a traditional form of Chinese bodywork that combines massage with some of the principles of acupuncture. By applying pressure to particular points on the body, the therapist aims to correct the flow of energy, or *qui*, which runs through invisible channels known as meridians. Using pressure to help relieve pain is one that is almost instinctive. Acupressure is useful in treating pain and stiffness in general, and trigger points in particular.

Suspected trigger point involvement

If your back pain has no cause, such as strain or arthritis, and persists, suspect trigger points. Research into chronic pain shows trigger points are often the cause of pain which does not rapidly get better on its own.

Lower back pain is often associated with triggers on the outer border of the large muscles near the spine, at waist level (quadratus lumborum). Pain in the leg, particularly down the back of the leg, is associated with triggers in the muscles of the buttock (gluetei), particularly those just under the rim of the pelvic bones.

Locating trigger points

Carefully search with your fingertips through muscles that are sensitive to find areas which, when pressed, cause pain—most usually a ache—to appear somewhere else in your body. These are trigger points.

Self-treatment of trigger points

Trigger points can be successfully treated using pressure or counterstrain and stretching.

Pressure

The point can be "deactivated" by applying direct pressure with your fingers or thumb or, if the point is not easily reached, a tennis ball.

- Using your thumb and forefinger, apply enough pressure to the muscle containing the trigger point so you can just feel pain in the target area. Hold this for about ten seconds before easing off. Do not let go of the place, but do not apply any pressure for another five seconds. Repeat ten seconds of pressure followed by five seconds rest for up to two minutes. Stop as soon as the pain in the target area starts to lessen as you reapply pressure after one of the rest periods.

- If the trigger point is not easily reached by hand (such as if located in the lower back), lie on a carpet and place a tennis ball under your back, easing your weight on to the ball in order to press the point. Use the same pattern of pressure and rest described above.

Below: If the trigger point is in the lower back, lie on a carpet and place a tennis ball under your back. Ease your weight on to the ball to apply pressure to the point for a minute or so, using a pattern of 10 seconds pressure and 5 seconds rest.

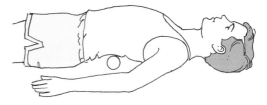

Counterstrain

Counterstrain methods, rather than pressure, can be used to deactivate the trigger point.

- Press the trigger point hard enough to produce both local and target-area discomfort. Then try to find a position which eases local and referred pain considerably. This usually happens as you bend toward the pain, twisting sideways one way or the other. When doing this, it is vital to make sure no new pain is produced. Once you find a position of ease, in which pain from pressure is greatly reduced, stay there for one minute.

Stretching

In order to deactivate a trigger point completely, it is essential to stretch the muscle in which the trigger point is situated painlessly. If this is not done, the trigger is likely to become active again very rapidly.

Place the muscle in which the trigger point lies at a painless stretch. This can be done by sitting and bending in one direction or another, by draping yourself over a folded cushion or by placing a limb at a stretch. The aim is to cause the muscle to be increased to a greater length, but without causing pain or stress.

TRIGGER POINTS

1 Lower trapezius
Trigger points in this muscle refer pain to the side of the neck, the upper aspect, and the back of the shoulder. They are often present and involved when shoulder movement is restricted and painful.

3 and 4 Multifidus
Multifidus comprises a series of "strips" which attach to the spine, helping to stabilize it. The upper multifidus point (just above the waist near the spine) refers pain around itself and to the abdomen on the same side. The lower multifidus trigger (near the base of the spine) refers pain to the low back, buttocks, and hip area. Both triggers may be involved in lower back conditions characterized by stiffness and spasm.

2 Levator scapula
Triggers in this muscle, which stabilizes the shoulder blade, affect the side of the neck, the shoulder and shoulder blade areas. Weakness or tightness may develop in the affected muscles causing the head to be carried to one side.

Referred pain from trigger points 3 and 4.

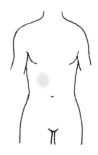

59

CHAPTER FIVE

RELAXATION TECHNIQUES

Because a great deal of emotional tension can be locked into our muscles, exercises which achieve "whole-body" relaxation are beneficial. The following progressive muscle relaxation and Autogenic training exercises achieve this and will help to prevent habitual tension.

PROGRESSIVE MUSCLE RELAXATION

The breathing exercises on pages 40-41 should always be performed before carrying out the exercises on these pages, because they prepare you for relaxation by calming the mind and reducing the activity of the sympathetic nervous system.

Progressive muscular relaxation

Wear loose clothing, lie on a carpet or rug, and make sure there are no drafts, and that you are unlikely to be disturbed for about 20 minutes.

1) Lie comfortably, arms and legs outstretched.

2) Tense the fist of your dominant hand and hold this tightly for about ten seconds.

3) Release the tension and stay like this for about 30 seconds, enjoying a feeling of heaviness.

4) Repeat this same muscle tension (dominant hand) at least once more, then rest "at ease" for 30 seconds.

5) Now do the same to the other hand (at least twice).

6) Now go to the foot on the side of your dominant hand. Draw the toes upward toward the knee, and hold for ten seconds.

7) Release and relax for half a minute and then repeat at least once more before going to the other foot.

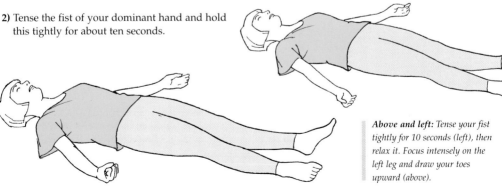

Above and left: Tense your fist tightly for 10 seconds (left), then relax it. Focus intensely on the left leg and draw your toes upward (above).

Perform this sequence in five other sites, such as:

- back of lower legs by pointing toes instead of drawing them up;

- upper leg, by pulling kneecap toward the hip;

- buttocks, by squeezing them together;

- chest/shoulders, by holding an inhaled breath and at the same time drawing shoulder blades together;

- abdominal area, by pulling in strongly;

- arms and shoulders by drawing upper arm into shoulder strongly;

- neck area, by drawing it into the shoulders or pushing it against the floor.

Always avoid any tightening which causes pain. The process of holding tightness, followed by release of this tightness, will give you an awareness of what tension feels like, because you will have regained a point of reference, something to compare it with.

After a week or so of doing this daily (twice daily is most beneficial if you can find the time) you can start to combine muscle groups, so your entire hand and arm on both sides can be tensed and then relaxed together; followed by your face and neck; then your chest, shoulders and back; and finally your legs and feet.

After another week of practice the tension element of the exercise can be abandoned altogether. You can simply lie down and focus on the different regions of the body one by one, noting whether or not they are tense, and instructing them to relax. Results come quickly, but only if the exercise is performed regularly!

Alternative relaxation exercise: modified Autogenic training

Every day, do the following for ten minutes:

1) Lie on the floor in a comfortable position, with one small pillow under your head and one under your knees, eyes closed. Do one of the breathing exercises on pages 40-44 for a few minutes.

2) Focus attention on your dominant arm and say to yourself "My arm feels heavy."

3) Try to sense the arm relaxed and heavy. "Feel" its weight. Over a period of about a minute silently repeat the sentence several times, and try to stay focused on the arms weight and heaviness. Your mind may wander but don't feel angry, just go back to the arm and its heaviness.

4) After a minute or so, focus on your left hand and arm, and repeat the exercise. Then repeat the exercise with your left leg, then your right leg.

5) Go back to your right hand and arm and this time tell yourself that you sense a greater degree of warmth there. "My hand is feeling warm."

6) After a minute move on to the left hand and arm, then the left leg and finally the right leg, each time with the "warm" message. If you sense warmth, stay with it and feel it spread. Enjoy it.

7) Finally focus on your forehead. Tell yourself it feels cool. Stay with this cool and calm thought for a minute before completing the exercise.

8) Finish by clenching your fists, bending your elbows and stretching out your arms.

ICE MASSAGE, HYDROTHERAPY, ESSENTIAL OILS

Ice Massage

To ease acute pain there are few more simple and effective methods than the application of cold. Most people think of heat as offering relief; however, all heat does is to draw more blood into an area which is usually already congested with acute back pain. After the first sense of ease, the area is likely to be even stiffer and more uncomfortable. Cold, on the other hand, decongests as well as having a painkilling effect.

There are a number of simple ways of applying cold safely:

- A bag of frozen peas (easily molded to the shape of the part being treated) straight from the freezer, wrapped in a hand towel and applied to the painful area for ten minutes every hour

- Commercially produced packs for use as cold applications (available from specialist stores, sporting goods stores, or drug stores)—use as above.

- A frozen hand towel (moisten and place in freezer)—lightly rinsed under cold water to make it flexible, applied as above (ten minutes per hour)

- An empty soft drink can, three quarters filled with water, and frozen. Remove it from freezer, seal the opening with tape and roll the can slowly over the painful area for three to five minutes per hour. The metallic cold transfers and absorbs heat more efficiently than the other methods, so avoid leaving the cold metal in one place. Keep it moving.

After any of the above methods, gently, carefully and without pain, ease, move and lightly stretch the tissues which have been chilled. Repeat every hour if possible until acute pain eases.

Hydrotherapy

The use of water can be effective in safely treating painful areas. This trunk-pack method has no contraindications and is useful in either acute or chronic stages of back pain.

Materials needed include:

- One or two thicknesses of cotton (tear up an old sheet) wide enough to reach from your underarm to your pelvis and long enough to pass just once around your body without overlapping.

- One thickness of wool or flannel material, a little wider and a little longer than the cotton so that a small overlap is achieved when it is used to cover the cotton. None of the cotton material should have access to air.

- Safety pins and cold water.

- A warm room in which to lie for several hours or as long as is necessary.

Run cold water over the cotton material (one thickness only at first) and ring it out so that the material is just damp, not dripping.

Wrap the damp material around your trunk so it covers you from the underarm to the pelvis. Immediately cover it with the wool or flannel, pinning it firmly so it completely covers the damp cotton, without any damp edges protruding. Lie down and cover yourself with a warm blanket.

This method can be used for just a few hours during the day, or overnight if necessary.

What should happen?
Within about five minutes any sense of cold should vanish and the material should feel comfortable. If it still feels cold after five minutes take the compress off and warm yourself.

After about 20 minutes the compress should start to feel hot. This should be maintained for several hours until it "bakes" itself dry.

The initial cold has a decongesting effect, followed by a neutral stage (same temperature as your body), which relaxes the muscles, followed by a period of damp warmth which enhances this relaxation.

If you have a strong constitution, good vitality and are not adversely influenced by cold, you could use two thicknesses of cotton, following all the same guidelines, for an even stronger effect.

Use this method three or four times weekly (alternate days) during either acute or chronic stages of back pain.

Make sure you wash the cotton material thoroughly before reusing as it will absorb acid wastes from the body which can irritate the skin.

Right: After about 20 minutes the compress should start to feel hot. This should be maintained for several hours until it "bakes" itself dry.

Aromatherapy oils
Essential oils are derived from different parts of plants—flowers, leaves, berries stems and roots. For use in a bath, no carrier oil is needed; simply place around 10 drops of essential oil into the water as the bath is running. For massage, add five drops of essential oil to an egg-cupful of a carrier oil (almond is ideal). Buy oils from a reputable supplier and store in a cool, dark place. Ideal oils for backache include:

- Camomile: one of the gentlest and most soothing of all oils. It is a natural anti-inflammatory, a successful analgesic, and a nerve sedative. It safely and naturally relieves tired, aching muscles.

- Rosemary: an effective antispasmodic and analgesic, rosemary is also very helpful for muscle ache.

- Eucalyptus: a natural analgesic, eucalyptus has the added bonus of being antiseptic. It mixes well with rosemary oil.

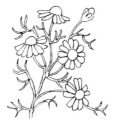

Left: Ideal oils for backache include Camomile (seen here) Rosemary and Eucalyptus.

CHAPTER SIX

COMPLEMENTARY CARE AND TREATMENT

Although most people with back problems first consult their medical advisors, few doctors are trained to deal with such problems. Modern research has shown that skilled manipulation for back problems eases pain and leads to a quicker recovery, compared with people receiving standard medical care or bed rest. An increasing number of back-pain sufferers are now choosing to receive attention from complementary health-care providers, such as osteopaths, chiropractors, massage therapists, and acupuncturists. Safe and effective treatment have been developed by these professions.

OSTEOPATHY AND CHIROPRACTIC

Osteopathy and chiropractic look at the muscles, ligaments and joints of the body—especially of the spine. When these are not working properly and/or are painful, they use specialized manipulation and rehabilitation techniques. Osteopathy and chiropractic differ from each other, as do both these systems from physical therapy, in their methods and philosophy. However, all three have borrowed ideas and techniques from each other and are now often difficult to tell apart.

What osteopaths and chiropractors believe

- The body is self-healing, given the chance. When structural and mechanical factors obstruct these self-healing tendencies, osteopathic and chiropractic treatment try to restore normal function.

- Any change in structure reduces functional efficiency. For example, a round-shouldered posture (structure) prevents free and deep breathing (function). Treatment aims at freeing those mechanical restrictions which prevent the normal breathing, at the same time as relieving discomfort associated with tight muscles and joints caused by this postural habit. The person is taught to stand and breathe better to prevent reoccurrence.

- Any habitual alteration in normal function eventually produces structural change. For instance, regularly wearing high heels throws the entire body out of line. The back muscles and joints become tense, stiff, achy, and,

Below: Osteopaths who manipulate pay attention to the soft tissues as well as to the joints. In this example, the osteopath is gently stretching the back muscles to relax these before performing mobilizing techniques.

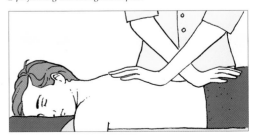

eventually, painful. Treating these changes helps to normalize them so that correct posture becomes possible again.

- The musculoskeletal system—muscles, fascia (a connective tissue lying beneath the skin and between muscles) ligaments and bones— is the body's largest energy user. Chronic stress of muscles and joints leads not only to problems such as back pain but also also to energy being wasted, resulting in fatigue. Osteopathic and chiropractic techniques can relieve such problems.

Diagnosing musculoskeletal problems
Apart from normal medical diagnostic methods, (chiropractors use X-rays), diagnosis is by physical examination and observation. In particular:

- Changes in the symmetry of the body, such as the different strength or length of muscles when one side is compared with the other.

- Restrictions or changes in the quality and range of joint movement compared with what is considered normal or with the same joint on the other side.

- Poor muscular coordination, and muscles being used by the body when they are not meant to be used.

- Changes in the texture of soft tissue because of:

overuse—repetitive movements in sport or work such as keyboard use
misuse—for example, awkward bending while gardening or in work settings
abuse—injury caused by falls, car accidents or other sudden events
disuse—insufficient exercise or function

Osteopathy and chiropractic try to restore normal tissue status, and to re-educate the person into better patterns of use. If more serious, underlying disease, such as arthritis, is suspected, an X-ray or scan is used to accurately diagnose this.

Despite focusing their therapeutic methods on the musculoskeletal system, both osteopathy and chiropractic are holistic, taking account of the whole person, their emotions, nutritional status, inherited factors and past medical history, as well as habits affecting the muscles, joints and bones.

Manipulative treatments
After taking a full case history and having performed an extensive musculoskeletal evaluation, an osteopath would have an insight into the complex, interacting factors that are producing the patient's symptoms. Problems with joints in the spine and disk changes that may result from them are a major feature of many forms of backache. However, most osteopaths consider the soft tissues—that is, muscles, ligaments and tendons— to be the prime culprits in creating back pain, since they determine the position of the bones.

Below: The chiropractor's hand is normalizing a neck restriction by moving the joint extremely quickly for a very short distance ("high velocity/low amplitude"), just as you might release a jammed drawer.

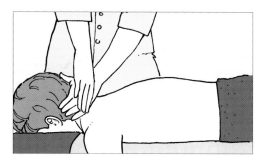

HERBAL, HOMEOPATHIC, AND NUTRITIONAL APPROACHES

Herbal medicines

While many herbal substances have been used for treating pain, few have been researched and found to be effective (although we should remember aspirin derives from a herbal extract of willow bark). Being more natural than many synthetic drugs does not make herbs safer to use. Indeed, some are undoubtedly toxic if overused.

- Pepper (cayenne): This causes the release of a chemical involved in the pain process (known as substance P) rendering it less potent after a short while. Rubbing cayenne pepper extracts onto chronically painful areas reduces pain after an initial reddening of the area. This is usually marketed with the word capsicum in the name and is not suggested for acute pain problems.

- Bromelain: If inflammation is present in a back-pain problem, as is almost always the case with an injury or strain, anti-inflammatory tactics are a useful aid to pain relief. We need to remember always the process of inflammation is itself is a part of the way the body heals injury, so we should not try to remove the inflammation altogether, just to reduce it sufficiently to make it tolerable. One of the safest ways of doing this is to take an extract of the pineapple plant, bromelain. This is an enzyme (minute chemical substances which take part in all body processes) which acts to ease inflammation and can be safely taken by anyone who is not sensitive or allergic to pineapples. The correct dosage is 500 milligrams taken four or five times daily away from mealtimes. If you take it with food it will help to digest the protein in your food (bromelain is a useful digestive) but will not then be available to calm the inflammation.

Dietary tactics

1) Reduce animal fats. Pain and inflammation involve prostaglandins and leukotrienes. Your body makes these from arachidonic acid, mainly derived from animal fats.

- Use fat-free or lowfat milk, yogurt, and cheese. Avoid butter altogether.

- Avoid meat fat completely and, if possible, eat a vegetarian diet for a time (or permanently). Avoid poultry skin.

- Look for and avoid hidden fats in products such as biscuits and manufactured foods.

2) Avoid instant coffee! Instant coffee blocks the receptor sites used by our natural painkilling endorphins, making pain seem more intense.

3) Eat fish or take fish oil. Fish from cold water areas such as the North Sea contain high levels of eicosapentenoic acid (EPA), which reduces arachidonic acid levels. You should:

- Eat fish such as herring, sardine, salmon, and mackerel at least twice weekly.

- Alternatively take 10-15 EPA capsules daily when inflammation is at its worst, then a maintenance dose of six daily.

4) Two to three grams daily DL-Phenylalanine has painkilling potential.

Homeopathic remedies

Homeopathy uses minute amounts of substances which in larger doses would induce symptoms very similar, or identical, to those which are present. Because of their extreme dilution homeopathic remedies are very safe, with no danger of a toxic reaction. They can be safely used even by pregnant women.

Listed here are the main remedies which may be useful for back pain. Some of them have recently received medical approval in stringent trials. Rhus. Tox, for example, was found to be effective in treating muscular pains and inflammations, as homeopaths have known for over a century.

Note: The letters and numbers following the name of the remedy indicate the degree of dilution ("potency") used. It is important to use not only the named substance but also its correct potency and dosage.

Cautions

- Homeopathic medication should be taken until improvement is noticed and then stopped until either there is no further improvement or the condition worsens again.

- It is important to avoid the use of rubs, ointments, and so on, of strong-smelling substances (such as camphor and wintergreen) when using homeopathic remedies.

- Homeopathic remedies should be correctly stored, in a cool dark place away from any fumes or aromatic smells.

- The remedies should be allowed to dissolve under the tongue, away from meal times.

THE MAIN REMEDIES

These are some of the main remedies for back pain. Use the remedy which most closely matches your symptoms.

Arnica 6X: Following accidents or injury, take a pill under the tongue every half hour until better.

Arnica 3X: Following bruising take one or two under the tongue every half hour.

Rhus Tox 6X: Take every hour when muscular pains ("fibrositis"/fibromyalgia) are strong. The pains of rhus tox are worse in cold, damp weather, like much arthritic pain.

Bryonia 6X: This is good for pain which is worse every time you move.

Below: Some homeopaths give their prescribed remedy to the patient at the end of a consultation. Remedies can be in liquid, pill, or powder form. A qualified homeopath has a range of remedies and chooses the one which best suits the individual.

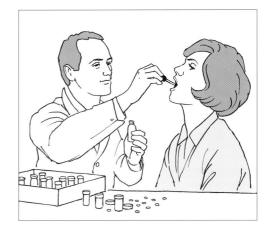

MASSAGE, ACUPUNCTURE, REHABILITATION

Soft-tissue Manipulation

A number of treatment methods have emerged from different disciplines such as osteopathy and chiropractic. These, in turn, have been successfully adopted by many other bodyworkers, including massage therapists, aromatherapists and physical therapists.

These methods include positional-release techniques and muscle-energy techniques, the self-help aspects of which have already been described (pages 42-45).

A number of other soft-tissue manipulation methods also deserve a mention in this section. These include Neuromuscular Therapy (also known as Neuro-Muscular Technique). This treatment focuses on locating and treating the myofascial trigger points (see pages 58-59), a major cause of back pain.

Other soft-tissue approaches to consider include craniosacral therapy and myofascial release methods, which target different soft tissues (muscle, ligament, tendon, fascia, and joint capsules) in treating back (or other) pain.

Since many of these methods are taught in short weekend courses, it pays to ensure that the therapist consulted is fully and properly qualified, licensed (in areas where this is a legal requirement to practice) and fully insured for professional liability.

Practitioners such as Rolfers and Heller Workers have had an extensive and lengthy training and will utilize many of these different methods to achieve improved posture and the most effective realignment of the body.

Acupuncture

The ancient Chinese methods of acupuncture have now become widely available in Western countries. Acupuncture is a major ingredient in traditional Chinese medicine, a sophisticated system of care which also includes herbalism, massage, diet, and exercise such as tai chi and chi gung. While some of the ideas surrounding acupuncture for general health problems remain controversial, there is little doubt that the use of needles can dramatically reduce pain. The ways acupuncture works have to an extent been explained in scientific terms, which makes it less difficult for doctors to accept, and many doctors now also use acupuncture in a limited way for certain conditions.

Traditional acupuncturists would want to take a detailed case history and treat each person individually taking into account all their symptoms, and looking at diet and emotional well-being as well. They would also assess the person's state of health by examining the tongue and taking the person's pulses. There are six, three on each wrist, and there are up to 28 pulse qualities.

Fine needles are placed (usually absolutely painlessly) into specific "points" based on the thousands of years of experience which the Chinese have accumulated in treating pain and disease in this way. The needles may be left in place for anything up to 20 minutes or may be removed quite quickly; they may be stimulated by electricity or by being gently rotated; or they may be heated by holding a hot source near the end of the needle. All these methods have different results, but they are seldom uncomfortable and are usually very successful in reducing pain.

Many bodywork therapists use these same-points by applying deep thumb or finger pressure into them, to achieve a similar result to that gained by needling (see pages 58-59).

MASSAGE AND SELF-MASSAGE

Traditional Swedish massage has expanded to incorporate a great many methods, such as the soft-tissue methods. It is now used to treat a wide range of both physical and emotional problems, including back pain and dysfunction. A variety of standards of training are required in different countries and states. Before consulting a therapist, check how extensive their training has been. Many therapists now treat sports injuries.

Self massage can help relieve tense muscles. Start by slowly and rhythmically lifting and circling the area with the whole hand. Squeeze painlessly, like wringing water out of a towel. Use fingers and thumbs to "work" tense areas painlessly.

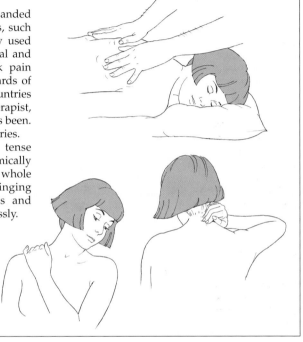

Right: Use the whole hand to stretch the muscle. Far right: Use fingers and thumbs to "tease out" tense muscles around the base of the neck. Above right: Start with light, gliding movements. Unless trained in massage, do not dig into painful areas.

Rehabilitation

Once the acute phase of a back problem is over, whatever treatment methods have been used to help lessen the pain programs such as those taught in Alexander Technique, Feldenkrais training, or Pilates (see pages 70-73) are useful in helping to learn new and safer ways of using the body, often remedying years of poor posture and bad habits such as sitting awkwardly or breathing dysfunctionally.

This rehabilitation phase is also a focus of attention for other professionals, including physical therapists and most osteopaths and chiropractors.

All these professionals employ slightly different variations on the same theme—exercises to help to reeducate function (how the person uses their body) as a way of preventing recurrence of the back problem.

It is vital for anyone who has experienced the agony, immobility, and frustration of back pain to take heed of this stage, and to work diligently at whatever program of exercise is prescribed, if they are to avoid a recurrence.

ALEXANDER TECHNIQUE AND YOGA

There are a wide variety of training, prevention, rehabilitation, and treatment systems. Space does not allow more than a brief discussion of some of the most beneficial of these.

Alexander Technique

The Alexander Technique (A.T.), based on the work of Australian F. M. Alexander (1869-1955) has emerged over the past century as an excellent way of relearning how to use the body in an efficient and unstressed way.

Efficient in this context means using just as little energy as is needed for any particular task, rather than wastefully using enormous amounts of physical effort where small amounts would do just as well. This reduces wear and tear on the joints and muscles, as well as saving energy.

Equally important is learning how to move, stand, walk, and generally function in the most unstressful (to the body) manner possible. A.T. is above all an educational experience, not a form of therapy and lessons are needed, either on a one-to-one basis or in small classes to help the relearning of good postural habits.

It is quite useless to tell someone who carries themselves in a posturally stressful way to "stand up straight." We have no internal guidance mechanism which tells us what straight is. All that is likely to happen when such instructions are given is that the person will stand badly in a different way.

Progress toward better posture comes slowly, as the A.T. teacher guides you into better use of the body, working on simple processes such as getting up and sitting down. Each person is treated as an individual.

A.T. has shown that if the head and neck can be held "correctly"in relation to the rest of the spine, much of the strain in the musculoskeletal system vanishes.

Arriving at an awareness of where the head and neck should be, and keeping it there effortlessly during everyday activities is the struggle involved in A.T. training, and it can take months of regular lessons to achieve this.

A.T. experience

- Stand in front of a chair. Place one hand behind your neck, holding it with the fingers curling toward the front to see what your neck does.

- Now sit back onto the chair but pay particular attention to what happens to your neck. Almost certainly you kinked your neck backward, poking your chin forward as you sat down. Did you feel this?

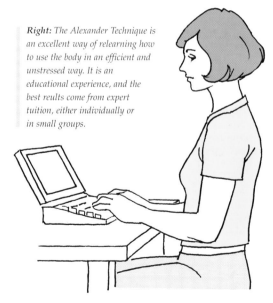

Right: The Alexander Technique is an excellent way of relearning how to use the body in an efficient and unstressed way. It is an educational experience, and the best reults come from expert tuition, either individually or in small groups.

- Now get up, still feeling your neck. Once again you kinked your neck and poked your jaw forward, didn't you?

- Try once more to accomplish these tasks, making an effort to lengthen your neck

when sitting down. As you begin to sit, bend forward from the waist, lengthen your neck and back, and plant yourself on the seat. This was less stressful. Try lengthening (still feeling your neck) as you get up again. A.T. training helps you relearn good habits.

Yoga

Traditional Indian medicine (Ayurveda) has among its many treasures the practice of yoga. This involves a comprehensive system of breathing and exercises in which postures (asanas) are adopted which stretch and tone all the muscles of the body, as well as influencing circulation and internal organ function, facilitating better health and wellbeing.

From the point of view of back problems, there are now advanced yoga teachers who practice yoga therapy. They can prescribe specific postures to be regularly practiced at home, in order to meet the needs of almost any spinal condition.

Yoga experience

This exercise, which is based on the "plow" yoga position, should not be attempted without prior evaluation of your condition by a health-care professional. Among other things, it is designed to stretch the whole spine as well as the backs of the legs.

Right: Do not attempt this exercise without first consulting your healthcare professional. It is based on a yoga position, and is designed to stretch the whole of the spine and the backs of the legs.

1) Lie face up on the floor, arms at your sides. Breathe in deeply and, as you exhale bend both knees onto your abdomen, straighten them toward the ceiling and take them backward over your head, using your hands to assist if necessary. Be careful to go straight back over your head and not over on one side.

2) Rest your toes on the floor behind your head, arms stretched out slightly sideways for balance. You should be aware of a stretch along your entire back as well as the backs of the legs.

3) Hold this position for a full minute, breathing deeply and slowly, before returning to the start position. Rest for a few breaths before rolling on to your side and sitting up.

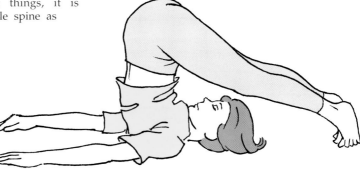

BIOFEEDBACK, TENS AND PILATES

Biofeedback

Biofeedback involves learning to alter a basic body function, or sign, using a machine which records this and displays it. It is possible for the individual to learn, for example, to modify their blood pressure, electrical resistance of the skin, or pulse rate, and in so doing achieve profound relaxation and changes in body function. Pain can be modified in this way as well.

Biofeedback is best learned from an expert such as a physical therapist who works in pain or rehabilitation medicine, or from a doctor who is experienced in its use.

It is not easy to teach yourself without such assistance. Success needs determination, patience, and the right sort of machine to give the information you need. Failure is usually due to lack of persistence or to difficulty in relaxing.

It is often useful to learn breathing and relaxation methods before starting biofeedback, which then allows deeper relaxation. The most successful area of pain control using biofeedback relates to headache, with the success rate rising when biofeedback is combined with autogenic training (see page 61). Improvements usually continue long after (for at least a year) the active use of biofeedback methods stops.

Other areas of pain which have shown a similar success rate to headaches include: neck muscle spasm, arthritis, TMJ problems (jaw) and pain following trauma.

A variety of inexpensive units exist which measure and display different sorts of information for biofeedback purposes. Those which measure the degree of tension in the muscles are thought to be the best for people with musculoskeletal aches and pains or tension-type headaches to use, as they encourage direct relaxation of the muscles.

TENS

TENS stands for transcutaneous electrical nerve stimulation. Tiny machines are carried in a pocket or purse, or are worn clipped to clothing, attached to two (or more) small pads which are placed strategically on the body.

A mild current passing through these pads can mask pain. TENS does not work on all pain; for example, it is relatively useless in treating inflamed nerve structures and very acute problems. It has a higher success rate when dealing with chronic pain. It is, however, very efficient in reducing most musculoskeletal pain if the pads are correctly sited, and the current correctly selected—most machines offer a range of current options.

There are no side-effects from TENS, and pain relief often lasts well after the use of the machine has ceased. These inexpensive machines are available to the public, but for best results seek the advice of a qualified health-care professional before starting to use them.

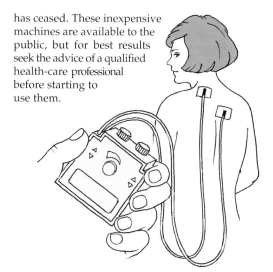

Pilates

Named after its German developer (Joseph Pilates, 1880–1967), this physical training and exercise method has been widely used for many years by people involved in the performing arts, notably dance, and by athletes. The general public has become slowly aware of the remarkable benefits of Pilates training, which is available at specialized gymnasiums in most large cities.

Pilates instructors require many years of training to become experts in analyzing the movement patterns of people attending for instruction. They prescribe a program of exercises, many of which involve the use of specifically designed apparatus. The rhythmic performance of these exercises is closely supervised to make sure that muscles are used correctly in a balanced manner, thereby reducing strain on joints and energy wastage.

The objective, of correct use of the body, is similar to that of the Alexander Technique (A.T.) but the methods employed in reaching the goals are very different. There are advantages to Pilates which go beyond A.T., since it offers a combination of suppleness and lengthening of muscles, as well as rebalanced activity, after regular application of the exercise program.

We noted on pages 20-21 how chain reactions of muscular imbalance can be a precursor of back problems, with some muscles becoming short and tight while others become weaker. When this happens compensations occur in which stronger muscles start to take over the roles of weaker ones. The problems which emerge can be quite complex as well as difficult to change. Pilates achieves change by encouraging muscles to work in their correct sequence. Repeating these sequences regularly helps the muscles to slowly relearn their normal activity.

The benefits of these changes to chronic back pain sufferers are obvious. What is even more important is that regular Pilates practice can prevent backache.

The illustration shows one of the more complex pieces of Pilates equipment called the "universal reformer" (not all the exercises require equipment and much can be done at home once the system has been learned).

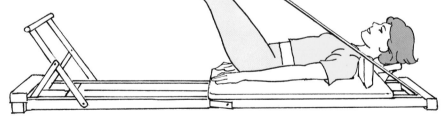

Left: A mild current passing through these pads can mask pain. TENS does not work on all pain; for example, it is relatively useless in treating inflamed nerve structures and very acute problems, and better in dealing with chronic pain.

Above: The illustration shows one of the more complex pieces of Pilates equipment called the "universal reformer." Not all the exercises need specialized equipment, and much can be done at home once the system has been learned.

USEFUL ADDRESSES

General Resources
UK
Back Pain Association
PO Box 780
London NW5 1DY

Acupuncture
USA
American Association of
Acupuncture and Oriental Medicine
4101 Lake Boone Trail, Suite 201
Raleigh,
NC 27607
(919-787-5181)

UK
British Acupuncture Association
37 Peter Street
Manchester
M2 5QD

Alexander Technique
USA
North American Society of Teachers of the
Alexander Technique,
PO Box 517, Urbana,
IL 61801
(800-473-0620)

UK
Society of Teachers of Alexander Technique
3B Albert Court
Kensington Gardens
London
W2 4RU

Biofeedback
USA
Association for Applied Psychophysiology
and Biofeedback
10200 West 44th Avenue, Suite 304
Wheat Ridge,
CO 80033
(303-422-8436)

Chiropractic
USA
American Chiropractic Association
1701 Clarendon Blvd.
Arlington,
VA 22209
(703-276-8800)

World Chiropractic Alliance
2950 N Dobson Road Ste 1
Chandler
AR 85224
(800) 347 1011

UK
British Chiropractic Association
120 Wigmore Street,
London
W1H 9FD

Feldenkrais
USA
The Feldenkrais Guild
PO Box 489
Albany,
Oregon 97321
(503-926-0981)

Massage

USA
American Massage Therapy Association
820 Davis St, Suite 100,
Evanston
IL 60201-4444
(708-864-0123)

UK
Fellowship of Sports Masseurs and Therapists
36 Lodge Drive
Palmers Green
London
N13

Osteopathy

USA
American Osteopathic Association
142 East Ontario Street
Chicago
IL 60611-2864
(312-280-5879)

American Academy of Osteopathy
3500 DePaauw Blvd. Suite 1080
Indianapolis,
IN 46268
(317-879-1881)

UK
General Osteopathic Council,
Premier House
10 Graycoat Place
London SW1P 1SB
(0171 799 2442)

Pilates

USA
Physical Mind Institute
1807 Second Street, #28129,
Santa Fe,
NM 87505
(505-988-1990)

UK
The Body Control Pilates Association
17 Queensbury Mews West
London
SW7 2DY
0171-581-7041

Rolfing

The Rolf Institute
P.O. Box 1868
Boulder,
CO 80306
(303-449-5903)

Yoga

USA
International Association of Yoga Therapists
109 Hillside Avenue
Mill Valley,
CA 94941
(415-383-4587)

UK
Yoga for Health Foundation
Ickwell Bury, Northill
Biggleswade,
Bedfordshire
SG18 9EF

Yoga Biomedical Trust
PO Box 140
Cambridge
CB4 3SY

INDEX